The Ethical Treatment of Depression

Philosophical Psychopathology: Disorders of the Mind
Jeffrey Poland and Jennifer Radden, Series Editors

The Ethical Treatment of Depression

Autonomy through Psychotherapy

Paul Biegler

The MIT Press
Cambridge, Massachusetts
London, England

© 2011 Massachusetts Institute of Technology

All rights reserved. No part of this book may be reproduced in any form by any electronic or mechanical means (including photocopying, recording, or information storage and retrieval) without permission in writing from the publisher.

For information about special quantity discounts, please email special_sales@ mitpress.mit.edu

This book was set in Stone Sans and Stone Serif by Toppan Best-set Premedia Limited. Printed and bound in the United States of America.

Library of Congress Cataloging-in-Publication Data
Biegler, Paul, 1963–
The ethical treatment of depression : autonomy through psychotherapy / Paul Biegler.
    p. ;   cm. — (Philosophical psychopathology)
Includes bibliographical references and index.
ISBN 978-0-262-01549-3 (hardcover : alk. paper)
1. Depression, Mental—Treatment—Moral and ethical aspects. 2. Cognitive therapy—Moral and ethical aspects. 3. Autonomy (Psychology) I. Title. II. Series: Philosophical psychopathology.
[DNLM: 1. Depressive Disorder—therapy. 2. Antidepressive Agents. 3. Cognitive Therapy—ethics. 4. Personal Autonomy. WM 171]
RC537.B487   2011
174.2'968527—dc22

2010036606

10 9 8 7 6 5 4 3 2 1

To the memory of my mother, Beryl Biegler

Contents

Series Foreword

The Philosophical Psychopathology series publishes interdisciplinary work that is broadly concerned with psychopathology and that has significance for conceptual, methodological, scientific, ethical, and social issues related to contemporary mental health practices, as well as for more traditional philosophical issues such as the nature of mind, rationality, agency, and responsibility. In providing a philosophical examination of the forms, limits, and lessons of mental disorder as well as its study and treatment, the broader goal is to foster an interdisciplinary community addressing issues about mental health and illness.

The present volume exemplifies the aims of the series in several respects. Its particular subject is depression, one of the most prevalent disorders throughout the world, and one that jeopardizes flourishing, health, and even life. Its prescriptive focus involves depression treatment, particularly the ethical imperative to prefer the autonomy-enhancing treatment modality of cognitive behavioral therapy. Biegler builds his argument here making use of equal parts theory, empirical studies, and the moral psychology of depression. Here are exhibited a firm grounding in science, including an understanding of cognitive psychology and of the psychopathology of depression; and attention to interfaces between basic science and the various cultural domains and issues found in the clinical context of depression treatment.

Biegler's argument, in brief, is that on a plausible, "epistemic" analysis of autonomy (autonomous choice as requiring justified beliefs about facts that are material to the individual, including facts about her affective responses), and given a preference for autonomy-enhancing treatment that is a norm within other biomedical practice, those treating depression and influencing health policy around its treatment have an ethical reason to choose cognitive behavioral treatment over other approaches. For in contrast to the alternatives, he argues, CBT teaches the individual to identify and challenge the unrealistic beliefs that negative biases foment.

This is a carefully researched and responsible piece of scholarly work. But it is more. The broader societal context—our "antidepressant" era, and the domination of pharmacotherapy in depression management— makes Biegler's work a call to arms. His aim, as he puts it, is to "prod the conscience of any physicians who believe their duty to those with depression is adequately discharged by simply writing a prescription for antidepressants."

The Ethical Treatment of Depression is an analysis with far-reaching impli- cations for practitioners and their patients, policy makers, and philoso- phers alike. Biegler has set the stage, we hope, for the kind of interdisciplinary exchange, collaboration and public debate over issues around mental health and illness that is the goal of this series.

Jeffrey Poland and Jennifer Radden, Series Editors

Acknowledgments

This book stems from my doctoral thesis, completed at the Centre for Human Bioethics at Monash University, Melbourne, Australia. I am indebted to my supervisors, Justin Oakley, Helga Kuhse, Nicholas Allen, and Ian Gold, for their invaluable assistance in the preparation of the thesis. I learned a great deal, both professionally and personally, through their advice and guidance. I am also deeply grateful to the postgraduate students of the School of Philosophy and Bioethics at Monash University for their comments during informal discussions and at seminar presentations of my work. In addition, the book has benefited from audience comments at the 2006 Australasian Postgraduate Philosophy Conference at the University of Tasmania and at the 2007 Australasian Association of Philosophy Conference at the University of New England, Armidale, New South Wales.

I owe special thanks to Dr. James Taylor of Sandringham Hospital in Melbourne and to the Alfred Health Network for the provision of sabbatical leave during which much of the preparatory work for the book was completed. I am also appreciative of financial support from a Monash Graduate Scholarship and a Monash Arts Postgraduate Publications Award. My father, Tom Biegler, has been especially helpful in proofreading and making comments on a manuscript draft.

Many thanks, too, are owed Jennifer Radden and Jeffrey Poland from MIT Press for their rigorous and enlightening critique, which has shaped several of the book's elements in its latter stages.

Finally, I thank Luci Renault and our beautiful children, Lydia, Adele, and Dylan, for sustaining me with their love and laughter, and for reminding me, regularly, that the book needed to be written.

1 Introduction

If you are not already sure that depression is a major global health issue, consider the following statistics. One in six people will experience depression over the course of a lifetime.[1] The incidence of depression is estimated to have increased from 50 cases per million people in the 1950s to 100,000 cases per million in the late 1990s.[2] In 2004, depression was the third highest contributor to the global burden of disease, at 4.3 percent.[3] In the same year, however, depression was the *leading* cause of disease burden in high- and middle-income countries, at 8.2 percent and 5.1 percent, respectively.[4] Greenberg estimates that depression cost the U.S. economy U.S. $83 billion in 2000, of which U.S. $26 billion comprised treatment costs and U.S. $52 billion represented workplace costs, including absenteeism and performance impairment.[5] To say these figures are disturbing risks serious understatement. However, statistics, even of this enormity, are still only a dispassionate measure of melancholy's reach. William Styron, a writer who experienced depression at first hand, gives a more intimate account:

[D]epression takes on the quality of physical pain. But it is not an immediately identifiable pain, like that of a broken limb. It may be more accurate to say that despair, owing to some evil trick played upon the sick brain by the inhabiting psyche, comes to resemble the diabolical discomfort of being imprisoned in a fiercely overheated room. And because no breeze stirs this cauldron, because there is no escape from this smothering confinement, it is entirely natural that the victim begins to think ceaselessly of oblivion.[6]

Styron's description makes plain why so many with depression are driven to seek relief through the health care system. In my own nation, Australia, about three-quarters of depression sufferers attend their general practitioner[7] and nearly 80 percent of those are treated with antidepressant medication (ADM).[8,9] In 2004–2005, Australian primary care physicians wrote over 11 million prescriptions for ADM, up from nearly 7.5 million in 1999–2000.[10] These are impressive numbers for a country whose population is a mere 22 million. The total cost of ADM prescriptions in general practice in 2004–2005 was just under half a billion Australian dollars, nearly double the amount of 1999–2000.[11] In the United States, the proportion of adults using ADM jumped from 2.5 percent in 1994 to 8 percent in 2002.[12] In that country, with a population of around 307 million, the number of ADM prescriptions rose from 154 million in 2002 to nearly 170 million in 2005.[13] Between 2000 and 2001 ADM sales in the United States increased from U.S. $10.4 billion to U.S. $12.5 billion, a rise of nearly 12 percent, cementing it as the highest selling drug category after cholesterol-lowering agents.[14]

It almost comes as a surprise, on viewing these figures, to learn that another, equally effective treatment for depression is available. Psychotherapy, in particular cognitive behavior therapy (CBT), has been subject to extensive trials that show its outcomes to be as good as those achieved with ADM. Ellis and Smith, funded by Australia's national depression initiative beyondblue, conducted a meta-analysis of 107 randomized controlled trials of depression treatment. In a summary that echoes national guidelines in the United States and the United Kingdom, they reached the following conclusion:

For the initial treatment, our meta-analysis shows there is little difference [in relative effectiveness] between the major pharmacological and psychological treatment options for mild to moderate depression.[15]

There is also emerging evidence that depressed people treated with CBT may have lower relapse rates compared to those who discontinue ADM after a successful response.[16] Despite this, in Australia less than a quarter of those who present to a general practitioner with depression will receive a validated psychotherapy, and figures in the United States are likely to be similar.[17]

In trials comparing CBT and ADM, treatment outcomes are commonly measured with the Hamilton Rating Scale for Depression.[18] It assesses the presence and severity of the typical symptoms of depression such as lowered mood, feelings of guilt, suicidal ideation, insomnia, anxiety, loss of energy or concentration, and indecision.[19] It also measures somatic symptoms such as reduced appetite, weight loss, or changes in bowel habit. There are several versions of the scale. The 21-item questionnaire has a maximum score of 66. A score of 12–16 indicates mild depression, a score of 17–23 indicates moderate depression, and score of 24 or greater indicates severe depression. For mild depression, neither ADM nor formal psychotherapy is necessary. Good results can be achieved with supportive counseling and problem-solving approaches, implemented with the aid of a primary care physician.[20] In moderate depression, ADM and psychotherapy, including CBT and interpersonal therapy (IPT),[21] are equally effective.[22,23] The same is true for severe uncomplicated depression,[24,25] that is, severe depression without associated psychotic features, medical illness, or substance abuse. As a result, Australia's beyondblue guidelines for the treatment of depression in primary care recommend that practitioners can use either psychotherapy or medication in these grades of depression.[26] Similar recommendations are made in the national guidelines of the United States[27,28] and the United Kingdom.[29]

Although ADM and CBT cause equivalent improvement in depression symptoms on Hamilton Rating Scale measures, there are obviously major differences between them. Most notably, pharmacotherapy can lift mood independent of any requirement that the patient *understand* prominent facets of his or her depressed response. In particular, the clinical effectiveness of ADM does not require knowledge of the action of lowered mood on thought processes or that psychosocial stressors can trigger depression.[30] On the contrary, this knowledge is essential for CBT, which teaches skills to deal with distressing feelings, negative thoughts, and causal stressors. Recommendations that the two treatments are equally effective and that, quite simply, either can be used fail to accord importance to these clear differences.

In this book, I show these differences to be critical and to form the basis for a profound ethical distinction between the two therapies. I argue the understanding gleaned through CBT concerns facts that are material to people with depression. As a result, I hold that personal autonomy is promoted through the therapeutic process. In contrast, ADM administered alone, I argue, affords no such understanding and so promotes autonomy in a different way and to a much lesser extent. I show that depression is a disorder in which patient autonomy is routinely and extensively undermined and that, as a consequence, physicians have a moral obligation to promote the autonomy of depressed patients. I conclude that an ethical imperative holds for medical practitioners to prescribe psychotherapy, and in particular CBT, for depression.

To begin, in chapter 2, I examine hierarchical, historical, life plan, and reasons-responsive theories to derive a meaningful construal of autonomy that forms a basis for the arguments to follow. I show that common to each theory is a view that autonomy is possessed by agents, free from serious constraints, who are equipped with resources adequate to enable actions that accord with deeply held values. I also note that serious disagreement exists on the precise properties of those desires that are possessed by autonomous agents. However, there is substantial concurrence that autonomous choice requires the agent to hold justified beliefs about facts that are material to the matter at hand. In refining an "epistemic" account of autonomy, I elaborate the nature of these beliefs, using the analogy of the informed-consent paradigm in medicine. I argue that a linear relationship holds between the number of material facts an agent grasps and the autonomy of his or her related decisions. I present this connection as a means of quantifying autonomy in depression, one with utility in the clinical context.

However, to ground the case for the moral obligation of practitioners to promote autonomy in depression, something must be said of why autonomy holds value, and the derivation of its normative force. To this end, I chart the rise of respect for personal autonomy as a guiding principle in medicine. I outline the attributes of autonomy that have fueled its recent prominence, over and against paternalism, in the physician–patient relationship. I highlight and explain the distinction, commonly drawn by philosophers, between the instrumental and intrinsic value of autonomy. I show that the normative force of autonomy derives from its capacity to further well-being, and from its association with personhood, a trait that confers moral status on the holder.

In chapter 3, I note that epistemic construals of autonomy have traditionally been concerned with beliefs about states of affairs that are external to the agent. For example, informed consent to surgery typically demands understanding of the incision site or the duration of the procedure. However, I switch the focus of material understanding inwards. Could accurate beliefs about one's emotional responses and psychological states also be important for autonomy? I answer this question in the affirmative, invoking three important facets of emotion in the process. First, I look at the evaluations integral to emotion. I argue that affective responses—those that entail "feelings"—provide evidence for the existence of characteristic triggering events and the value to the agent of their outcomes. The argument draws on "appraisal" theories suggesting emotions are set off by events that have critical implications for the agent's interests. Building on these accounts, I argue that facts about such events are material to the individual and that accurate interpretation of his or her affective response enhances the autonomy with which the agent addresses an emotive trigger. Two remaining facets of emotion add force to the argument. First, empirical evidence is adduced that emotion aids decision making and, indeed, might be essential for it. Second, emotion is shown to be a powerful motivator of behavior. I argue that emotion's profound influence on decisions and action makes a skilled grasp of its evaluative content crucial for autonomy.

In making this case I deal with the inescapable reality that emotions can, and do, mislead. Emotion can reflect misunderstanding and skewed perception and sometimes bears little relation to events in the world. Agents then layer their interpretation on emotions, sometimes accepting at face value those that are wrong-headed or, less commonly, ignoring those that accurately render reality. I argue that autonomy is undermined when the agent uncritically accepts, and acts on, emotions that wrongly report environmental events. To clarify this claim, I conceive the "evidential value" of affect. Roughly, evidence adduced in favor of a proposition raises the probability, for the agent, that the proposition is true. I note that affect typically reinforces the conviction with which agents hold related beliefs. Thus, I suggest the affective response provides some "evidence" to the individual for the truth of his or her associated beliefs. I then propose that affect with a tendency to reinforce justified beliefs be construed as having high evidential value. Conversely, affect that tends to strengthen unjustified beliefs possesses low evidential value. I argue that because affective appraisals pertain to material states of affairs, the agent who unwarily accepts beliefs primed by affect of low evidential value is prone to hold unjustified beliefs about material facts. As a result, the autonomy of the agent's resulting actions is diminished.

In chapter 4, I apply this concept to affective disorder, arguing that affect in depression has poor evidential value, that is, it tends to reinforce unjustified associated beliefs. I show that two processes underpin this effect. First, negative affect drives information-processing biases that lead to unrealistically pessimistic predictions concerning the object of the affective response. Second, I present data showing psychosocial stressors trigger around 70 percent of depressive episodes.[31] I detail studies that strongly suggest many depressed people do not appreciate a causal role for stressors. Further, I show that, even when stressors are identified, negative affect mediates a biased appraisal of them. I conclude that depressed people are unlikely to hold justified beliefs about negative biases and the role of psychosocial stressors in depression. I show this information to be material and that ignorance of it undermines autonomy.

I move on to compare how ADM and CBT address the autonomy lapses seen in depression. In chapter 5, the focus is on negative biases. I explain how CBT teaches the individual to identify and challenge the unrealistic beliefs that negative biases foment. I marshal empirical data supporting "debiasing" as integral to the mechanism of CBT. The unrealistic pessimism born of biased thinking is displaced, through CBT, by more reliable predictions, furthering autonomy. While acknowledging that ADM can also modify depressive pessimism, I argue that pharmacological debiasing is notably distinct, in two ways, from that achieved through psychotherapy. First, the person treated with ADM alone is denied an understanding of the negative biases associated with depressed affect. Because this understanding is material, ignorance works against personal autonomy. Second, depressed people treated with CBT appear to retain a facility to generate negative affect. However, for the person receiving ADM it seems a "floor" is put in place, below which affect cannot fall. Scope for negative affective swings is restricted by ADM. I argue, based on appraisal theory, that negative affect has utility as a marker of events that are material to the agent. The CBT-treated person, in virtue of his or her preserved capacity for negative affect, maintains an ability to identify events as material and, therefore, to flag them as meriting evaluation. I argue the ADM-treated individual is denied this opportunity and conclude that the person receiving CBT is more likely, as a result, to hold justified beliefs about materially significant affective triggers. Greater autonomy ensues for the recipient of CBT.

In chapter 6, I turn to the role of psychosocial stressors in depression. CBT invokes a problem-focused strategy to address stressors, an approach I show assists understanding of three salient facets of depression. First, depressive episodes are often brought on by stressors, and those stressors are typically bound to the depressed person's principal interests. Second, depression represents a maladaptive response to stressors, threatening the agent's related interests.[32] Finally, that dysfunctional response can be addressed through therapy in a way that protects the interests at stake. I show this broad category of information, and its peculiar content in the individual's circumstance, to carry material weight for the person with depression, whose autonomy is furthered through its understanding. Treatment with ADM alone furnishes no such understanding, grounding an autonomy advantage for those receiving CBT. I conclude that CBT promotes autonomy in depression to a greater degree than does ADM, but I concede that an obligation for physicians to prescribe CBT does not automatically follow.

In chapter 7, however, I present the case that medical practitioners are bound by a pressing moral obligation to recommend CBT in depression. I use "parity of reasoning" to argue that autonomy promotion through informed consent and through chronic disease self-management forms an ethical template supporting autonomy promotion through psychotherapy in depression. I then argue that the autonomy threat posed by depression, manifest in high rates of relapse and recurrence, makes the degree of autonomy promotion seen with CBT both a proportionate and a warranted response. I acknowledge that autonomy is one of a number of principles that might properly influence the treatment recommendations of doctors. However, after examining notions of the proper goals of medicine, professional autonomy, cost–benefit utility, and beneficence, I affirm that autonomy remains of paramount concern in treatment of depression.

I conclude that a forceful ethical obligation exists for practitioners to provide CBT for their depressed patients. My entreaty comes in a Zeitgeist where pharmacotherapy dominates depression management and only a substantial minority of patients receives CBT. If I am right, this imbalance is cause for grave concern, with doctors failing on a vast scale to uphold their ethical obligations to patients with depression. I allude to a number of factors that might perpetuate the high incidence of pharmacotherapy in depression, such as direct-to-consumer advertising and pharmaceutical company sponsorship of medical education. I also note that many doctors may be impeded in efforts to provide psychotherapy through circumstances beyond their control. These include inadequate remuneration of physicians who wish to deliver psychotherapy as well as limited access to appropriately trained psychologists. However, my case should strengthen the resolve of those frustrated by resource constraints to agitate for wider access to psychotherapy. It will also, I hope, prod the conscience of any physicians who believe their duty to those with depression is adequately discharged by simply writing a prescription for antidepressants.

2 Autonomy: The Importance of Justified Beliefs about Material Facts

In this chapter, I provide the account of autonomy that will inform claims that doctors are morally required to promote this trait in their depressed patients. I set out agency and liberty as foundational elements of autonomy and then elaborate four contemporary theories that stipulate the kinds of desires compatible with actions under full agential control. While accepting that autonomy requires actions to cohere with desires and values the agent endorses as his or her own, I argue that conceptual difficulties with desire-based theories limit their clinical utility. For this reason, I focus on the nature of the beliefs an agent must hold for his or her related actions to be autonomous. I argue that justified beliefs concerning material facts are necessary for autonomous choice and that autonomy can be quantified by enumerating those material facts that are fully understood by the agent. I go on to explain how autonomy accrues value on both instrumental and intrinsic accounts before showing that value to be a source of the normative weight accorded the principle of respect for autonomy. The view of autonomy presented here will be developed in the next chapter, where I argue that an understanding of the emotional response is central to a full account of personal autonomy.

2.1 Autonomy: Fundamental Principles and Four Contemporary Accounts

The term "autonomy" has its roots in the Greek *autos* meaning "self" and *nomos* meaning, "rule," "law," or "governance." The original usage of autonomy was as a descriptor for Greek city-states that were self-determining and not subject to the law or will of another state.[1] The notion of personal autonomy extends this earlier political conception to the individual. Thus, an autonomous individual can be thought of as someone who "governs" himself or herself, rather than being dictated to by another.

Those who are compelled always to act at the behest of others are not autonomous but heteronomous. As with political governance, individual self-governance emphasizes an overarching credo, plan, or set of values with which the actions of the individual cohere.

Most conceptions of autonomy embrace two elements, liberty and agency.[2] Isaiah Berlin has argued that liberty has both a negative and a positive sense.[3] In its negative sense, liberty implies freedom from external impediments to intentional action. Negative liberty is widely held to be a necessary condition for autonomy. Thus, the person who is imprisoned or enslaved, being paradigmatically unfree, is also deprived of autonomy. However, as Robert Young has pointed out, liberty in this negative sense is not sufficient for autonomy.[4] The slave does not become autonomous simply by virtue of being released from the bonds of slavery. If, for example, during bondage the slave became mentally or physically impaired, perhaps as a result of illness, then, although later free, he or she is not necessarily autonomous.

A fuller account of autonomy invokes the notion of positive liberty. It requires that individuals be assisted in achieving self-determination through the provision of appropriate resources. Consider a variation on Locke's case. A person is placed in a room believing its only door to be locked when in fact it is unlocked. In one sense the person is quite free to leave but in another sense is not. The person is "free" in a negative sense as there are no physical barriers to leaving the room. However, without knowing the door is unlocked, he or she is deprived of liberty in its more positive sense.[5]

Agency, the second broad requirement for autonomy, can be thought of as the capacity for intentional action.[6] The notion of agency conveys the sense of a power to act and implies an authority over oneself based on an ability to formulate plans and to carry them out. Agency demands a capacity to rationally process the information that grounds beliefs, desires, and ultimately, our motivations to act. A lack of agency is the primary contributor to the diminished autonomy of the freed slave with mental or bodily impairment. In recent decades four accounts have been particularly influential in further molding the concept of personal autonomy. Each has its foundation in notions of liberty and agency but attempts to refine, in particular, the kinds of desires that might form the basis for a satisfactory account of autonomy.

Hierarchical theories, proposed by Gerald Dworkin,[7] Harry Frankfurt,[8] and others,[9] are so named because they emphasize concordance between different "hierarchies" or tiers of desires as necessary for related actions to be autonomous. For example, a person addicted to drugs who also wants to be drug free experiences conflict between the first-order desire to use and the second-order desire to desist. On a hierarchical account, a failure to endorse the first-order desire at a higher level leaves the autonomy of the resulting action in doubt.

One criticism leveled at the hierarchical account is termed the "problem of authority."[10] In virtue of what property, the objection runs, ought "higher order" desires to be seen as emblematic of autonomy? What defining characteristic, for example, of the desire for drug abstinence makes it authoritative in determining autonomy? Gary Watson has framed the concern concisely:

Second order volitions are themselves simply desires, to add them to the context of conflict is just to increase the number of contenders; it is not to give a special place to any of those in contention.[11]

Hierarchical accounts are also termed "time slice" theories because they take a moment in time and examine the desires present at that reference point. John Christman pinpoints this aspect of the hierarchical approach as inadequate. Christman argues that it is how desires come about, rather than their properties at any given moment, which has most relevance for whether we deem the ensuing actions autonomous.[12] On his "historical" view, our motivating desires must arise through rational self-reflection and develop without resistance. Imagine a young swimmer, heavily influenced by parental expectations, who reluctantly attends early morning training sessions during his teenage years. On Christman's account, the aversion apparent during the pursuit of this sport, if a product of lucid reflection, suggests diminished autonomy in the motivations that later drive the swimmer's participation.

Christman's theory faces an important objection. Can't desires that arise freely and rationally also hamper autonomy? Alfred Mele posits the example of a middle-aged man who, as a student, cultivated a desire for hard work and achievement.[13] Now, he wishes to spend more time with his child but cannot banish the ingrained drive to succeed or the long working hours it entails. A desire that is initially autonomous on historical criteria seems to run counter to autonomy at a later time.

A third important approach to personal autonomy is that of Robert Young, who asks us to differentiate between the short-term interests that fuel many day-to-day decisions and the kinds of longer term goals that comprise a "life plan."[14] For Young, when we act to satisfy our quotidian concerns, we might demonstrate "occurrent" autonomy, or autonomy "of the moment." However, when we are guided by and conform to our overarching concerns, we evince "dispositional autonomy," an autonomy that has greater worth because it subserves goals that more fully reflect our deepest values. On this account, a professor who risks her marriage, family, and career in a one-night stand with a student might, in that situation, satisfy the criteria for occurrent autonomy. However, by frustrating goals of overriding importance, she acts at the expense of her dispositional autonomy and in a manner that is, ultimately, self-defeating. A question for this kind of account is how one adjudicates autonomy in the setting of a newer, alternative life plan. For example, the professor, fed up with the stress of academic life and the monotony of a loveless relationship, may have seriously considered embarking on an affair. It remains unclear on what basis we should give precedence to this radically altered plan, or the one it succeeds, when making assignations of dispositional autonomy.

John Fischer and Mark Ravizza have refined a "reasons-responsive" account of autonomy.[15] It proposes that the autonomous agent must be sufficiently aware of and sensitive to the main reasons for and against acting in a particular way. Reasons need to be recognized as strong or weak and must be correctly located on a continuum that orders them according to strength. Strong, or good, reasons are to be seen as more powerfully motivating than weak, or poor, reasons. Consider an elderly man who attends hospital with abdominal pain and is diagnosed with bowel cancer at an early stage when surgery is likely to be curative. The man refuses admission because he has scheduled an overseas trip to visit his ailing mother. On a reasons-responsive account, we should seriously question the autonomy of his refusal because, it seems, he is rejecting the option that he has most reason to pursue.

Yet, this example highlights a concern raised by John Christman, who argues that reason-responsiveness underplays the importance of our emotional commitments.[16] Can analysis of reasons adequately capture the emotional value we attach to seeing a much-loved relative? Does such an approach mean that actions stemming from passion or whim are simply inconsistent with autonomy?

These theories add refinements to both the liberty and agency conditions that govern personal autonomy. For example, it is plausibly a matter of liberty that individuals be able to form preferences in a manner free from pressure or undue influence, as specified in Christman's historical criterion. Also, if agency demands that the power to act derives from the *agents themselves*, accounts that elucidate which desires truly emanate from the self, such as hierarchical and life-plan accounts, further our under-standing of the agential requirements for personal autonomy. It follows, too, that a failure of agency manifests when individuals fall short of a reasons-responsive threshold for autonomy. To choose to be moved by weak rather than strong reasons suggests a rational lapse that is inconsis-tent with agential control.

This brief sketch only gestures at the substantial contribution to our understanding of autonomy made by each theory. However, the aim is not to detail these accounts in full but to acknowledge, even if only in outline, the broader notion of autonomy to which they refer. The discussion thus far shows autonomy to comprise a number of elements. Agency implies that individuals act with intention and that the locus of control for action derives from the agent himself or herself, not from some external source. A substantial goal of the four theories mentioned is to stipulate the nature of those motivating desires that belong to the agent, and whose expression is thus emblematic of agential rather than heteronomous control. It is, therefore, a requirement for autonomy that decisions and actions cohere with desires that are sanctioned by the agent. Negative liberty plays a permissive role, in that a necessary condition for autonomous action is freedom from serious impediments or constraints. Positive liberty demands more, by requiring additional resources to aid the individual in realizing both agency and autonomous choice.

While these theories add considerably to a coherent picture of auton-omy, it is evident that none, in present form, presents a framework allowing autonomy to be readily assessed in a clinical context. An inher-ent difficulty lies with the normative weight that each theory places on desires. This specification requires those charged with determining auton-omy to achieve consensus on a rational benchmark by which to evaluate desires. However, as the objections to each theory attest, desires are noto-riously resistant to this kind of rational adjudication. To ascertain auton-omy through reference to an individual's desires is to be prescriptive in relation to the properties and ultimately the content of those desires. But on what basis are we to prescribe a desire for another, whether it be to abstain from drug use, pursue a swimming career, see more of our chil-dren, or even undergo a life-saving operation? While we might appeal to the benefits and drawbacks of various options as reasons to favor or reject them, individuals will ultimately weight those utilities according to taste, something not easily measured by any objective parameter. Bernard Berofsky has formulated this challenge for autonomy theory in the following way:

If we come upon an agent with abhorrent, foolish, or outrageous desires, is there a rational procedure which can convince him to abandon those desires other than by showing him that they are based on false or improbable beliefs or that their pursuit would interfere with other goals of his? Current accounts of autonomy do not hold a great deal of promise in this regard.[17]

Moreover, setting aside conceptual concerns, there remain empirical difficulties with the kinds of evaluations called for by desire-based accounts of autonomy. Analyzing tiered desires for concordance, chronicling the genesis of a certain wish, discerning the degree of fit of short-term and long-term motivations, and examining the relative strength of various reasons are complex exercises unlikely to deliver consistent results in the consulting room.

If desires are relatively resistant to rational assessment, beliefs are far more compliant in this regard. Beliefs need to accurately reflect states of the world that, in the main, invite reasoned agreement. If I believe a length of fabric to measure ten yards, my belief can be proven to be true or false in a way that my liking for the material, or my desire to purchase it, cannot. Put another way, while we can, in many cases, converge on a correct view about the objects of belief, correctness seems not to apply to the objects of desire except in a way that is irreducibly contingent on prevailing social or moral norms. For example, a desire to run naked down the main street might seem, at first glance, irrational. Yet if the street were the temporary domain of a New Age festival that encouraged nudity, we might instead think the desire rational. In contrast, false beliefs about states of the world (such as the length of a piece of fabric) that persist in the face of incontrovertible contrary evidence signal irrationality even when contingent factors are varied. It is their more rigorous and measurable aspect that suggests beliefs as a promising yardstick by which to identify, and indeed to quantify, personal autonomy.

My object is to determine when, how, and to what degree depression undermines personal autonomy and to compare the relative effects of psychotherapy and ADM to promote autonomy in this disorder. Plainly, desires undergo major shifts in those with depression. The once-gregarious person can wish for nothing but solitude, the avid gastronome might lose all interest in food, and the lover of life could now wish for it to end. Moreover, a complete account of autonomy must specify some coherence between the agent's behavior and those desires, goals, or values that are most cherished, deeply held, or directly derived from the agent himself or herself. Yet, it is apparent that evaluating desires to make conclusions about autonomy is, at the very least, problematic both conceptually and empirically. As a result, I will not attempt to advance this part of the debate, and I will allude only broadly to the concordance between actions and values that is a condition of autonomy. While recognizing a desire-based framework as integral to a complete account, my focus will be restricted, for the reasons outlined, to the nature of those beliefs necessary for autonomy.

2.2 Epistemic Autonomy

Epistemology is the branch of philosophy concerned with defining knowledge and determining the nature of justified true beliefs. In this section I want to show how the holding of justified beliefs is important for autonomy. First, though, it is necessary to allude to some complexities. In particular, I want to briefly distinguish between "true" and "justified" standards of belief and explain why I will adopt the latter as the basis for the account of autonomy presented.

On a common definition, to have a belief is to hold a given proposition to be true. Plainly, I can be justified in holding true beliefs. For example, if I believe the time as it appears on a consistently reliable clock, it is likely that my belief about the time of day will be both justified and true. However, I can also be justified in holding false beliefs. If the same clock failed inexplicably, leading me to believe a time that was inaccurate, under the circumstances many would deem my belief justified, even if incorrect. Imagine, on the other hand, that I happened to glance and note the time on a child's toy watch that was felicitously set to the correct hour and that I mistakenly took the toy to be a working timepiece. In this case, I come to hold a true belief about the time, but without proper justification. This is an example of "epistemic luck." In such cases, many philosophers seriously question whether the resulting belief qualifies as knowledge.

In medicine, many beliefs do not arise from the contemporaneous evaluation of discrete objects but concern future medical procedures and possible outcomes of disease. It is apparent that an autonomy standard requiring true beliefs about these kinds of probabilistic future outcomes would frequently be too demanding. Take the example of someone consenting to routine hernia surgery who believes the result will be uneventful. Unfortunately, there is a postoperative deep venous thrombosis, a recognized complication of surgery that had been explained beforehand. Autonomy would mandate omniscience, or something approaching it, if true belief about this kind of occurrence were a prerequisite. Instead, it might seem more reasonable to require true beliefs about the probability or risk of complication. Yet even here true beliefs can be an exacting condition. What might be a "true" indication of risk at one time could be subject to later revision based on fresh data from, for example, a more comprehensive study. But a true belief standard can also, in some cases, fail to be demanding enough. If an accurate prediction resulted from "epistemic luck," it would lack sufficient rigor to form a criterion for autonomy. Imagine the hernia patient now suffers from dementia and holds beliefs about surgery that alternate according to the day of the week. One day the patient believes she will undergo heart surgery, and the next she correctly believes the operation will repair a hernia. If consent happened to be given on the "hernia day," while a true belief about the nature of surgery is evident, its dubious grounds give little cause to adduce autonomous consent based on that belief.

However, a justified belief standard is also problematic, most obviously because such beliefs can be false. The hernia patient (now cognitively intact) would seem to be justified in believing the surgeon will operate on the correct side, given the examination findings and the surgeon's exemplary track record. Yet, if the surgeon mistakenly operated on the healthy side, the patient's justified belief would be shown false and, given the importance of the object of belief, would seem to be inimical to the autonomy of her consent. A justified belief standard in this case seems unable to ensure autonomous choice.

Despite these difficulties, there remain reasons to favor a justified belief approach. On one view, to be justified in believing is to hold *adequate* grounds for belief, where "a belief has adequate grounds if it is statistically probable that a process of belief production from grounds of that kind will yield a true belief."[18] Therefore, on this definition, beliefs premised on adequate grounds have a greater than 50 percent probability of reflecting the truth. Implicit in this approach is that adequacy and justification admit of degrees, with stronger grounds leading to more justified beliefs, which, in turn, carry a greater likelihood of tracking truth than beliefs with less justification. It is further possible to specify varying standards for the necessary grounds. For example, a narrow standard might encompass only those facts of which the agent is immediately aware. A wider standard could include facts gleaned after a small amount of research. A very wide standard might specify all those facts "generally believed in the community."[19] I want to suggest that it is reasonable to adopt a requirement for justified beliefs based on wider grounds in that it avoids overly exacting standards of truth while being compatible with realistic expectations about how much can be known.

To illustrate, consider someone commencing a medication for high blood pressure. The treating physician gives a hurried assurance the new drug is compatible with the patient's other medications. The patient arguably forms a justified belief, on the grounds that a physician is the source of information, that there will be no unfavorable interactions between the new and existing medicines. Yet, in this instance, the overworked doctor has made an error and there is a risk of dangerous interaction, a risk explicitly detailed in the leaflet accompanying the drug. Moreover, the clinic has introduced a protocol requiring that all patients be reminded to read and heed product information, which the doctor in this case has ignored. Given the existence of this more rigorous standard, and the ready availability of drug information, it is dubious that a simple assurance by the doctor can be construed as adequate grounds on which to justify a belief. It is more plausible that a justified belief in this case would require consideration of the best available evidence to which the patient could reasonably be expected to have access. It is to this standard that I will refer when I use the term justified belief. This type of approach is consistent with that proposed by philosophers Faden and Beauchamp, who describe a justified belief as "the common sense conception of reasonable (even if not true) belief and assertion that underlies ordinary social agreements about what is veridical."[20]

A number of philosophers have noted the importance of justified beliefs for autonomy. John Benson, for example, states, "To be autonomous...is to put oneself in the best position to answer for the reliability of one's beliefs. It is to be in charge of one's epistemic life."[21] Benson stresses that "assessment of testimony" is a pivotal process for those who seek to hold justified beliefs. Benson's account likens the autonomous agent to a judge who must weigh the evidence presented in order to reach the truth. A common quandary is whether to accept the word of others or to verify information through personal appraisal. Thus:

It may well be the case that one's chance of possessing a justified true belief is greater if one makes no attempt to investigate the matter at first hand. This will obviously be true if one lacks expertise in the appropriate field, say anatomy, skill in diagnosis, experience in using a microscope, etc.[22]

However, if the testimony of others is vulnerable to bias or distortion, then it ought not to be accepted uncritically.

Should one eat butter? The experts who say "No" are funded by the margarine manufacturers; those who say "Yes" are funded by the Milk Marketing Board. The man of sense will ignore both.[23]

Robert Young also notes the importance for autonomy of an adequate appreciation of facts and an ability to rationally manipulate them:

Depending on the magnitude of their mistakes, those who draw invalid inferences or make use of incomplete or partially reliable information are likely to suffer in their overall autonomy from these failures in rationality.[24]

For Young, a sound epistemology is necessary to ensure that everyday behavior accurately interprets the agent's dispositional goals. Rationality, as he puts it, "brings coherence into the relationship between a person's general purposes and his or her particular actions."[25]

And Sarah Buss points out that ignorance, if it causes the agent who wishes to do x to instead do y, vitiates the authorization condition that is required for autonomous agency:

[I]f I have a general desire to do what is right and prudent...then insofar as I am moved to act in ways incompatible with satisfying those desires, there is a sense in which...I have not authorised my actions."[26]

These writers lay down some important epistemic ground rules for autonomy. In fields beyond the autonomous agent's ken, he or she should devolve responsibility for fact gathering to specialists, but the onus remains with the agent to verify the credentials of those whose testimonials are relied on. If one is to realize goals consistent with life plans, deliberative rationality must be brought to bear on complete and reliable data. Agency suffers when a failure of comprehension leads the individual to pursue a path in error. Yet, while these stipulations are broadly helpful, it remains unclear precisely what, of the plethora of relevant information, needs to be understood, and believed, for actions to be autonomous. What must the individual know to satisfy the requirements of agency, and positive liberty, to a degree that permits adequate autonomy to be deduced? One area where the role of beliefs in autonomous decision making has been closely scrutinized is the informed-consent paradigm in medicine. It forms a useful template with which to further examine the issue.

2.2.1   Autonomy and Justified Beliefs; the Model of Informed Consent

Consider the case of Gideon, a middle-aged writer who has experienced chest pain and seeks advice from a heart specialist. An angiogram demonstrates blockages in all three main coronary arteries. The specialist outlines two treatment options. Gideon can take medication which will control his chest pain, but only if he limits himself to minimal exertion, such as moving around the house. He will not be able to play tennis or jog, his favorite pastimes. The alternative treatment is coronary artery bypass surgery. While surgery has a high chance of success with mortality rates below 1 percent, it also carries an 80 percent chance of cognitive impairment, which is probably caused by the heart–lung bypass that is necessary in this type of operation. Cognitive deficits include reduced concentration, loss of memory, and a sensation that some describe simply as "not being the same."[27] If Gideon were so affected, then his ability to continue writing would be jeopardized. He understands the risks and benefits of each treatment, and the specialist asks him to choose.

How do beliefs contribute to the autonomy of Gideon's decision? It is plausible that justified beliefs about the effects of surgery will expedite a choice that reflects Gideon's cherished values. He is passionate about writing, which is also his livelihood. Bypass surgery presents a significant risk to his literary ambitions and to his source of income. On the other hand, sport and exercise, which will be restricted if Gideon opts for medication, are also important to him. After lengthy consideration Gideon concludes that his stronger wish is to write, and so he declines surgery, instead electing to control his symptoms with medication. Here, justified beliefs have been integral to a choice that will, it is hoped, preserve the capacities that Gideon most values.

However, if we disagree on whether autonomy is better explained by, for example, hierarchical, historical, life-plan, or reasons-responsive accounts, in what sense can we say that justified beliefs have contributed to the autonomy of Gideon's choice? Indeed, it is quite reasonable to see justified beliefs as important for autonomy under *each* of these formulations. For example, whatever desire is deemed definitive of autonomy on a hierarchical account, it is plausible that justified beliefs about suitable means will expedite its fulfillment. Implicit, too, in the requirement for rational self-reflection specified by John Christman, is the notion that a sound epistemology grounds historical autonomy. In addition, justified beliefs are integral to the successful matching of actions with overarching life plans and also to ensuring that guiding reasons are firmly based in reality. Justified beliefs are, therefore, very broadly applicable to the notion of autonomous action. However, the present concern—to compare the effect of ADM and psychotherapy on autonomy—requires a quantitative measure. Can we use beliefs to quantify autonomy? For example, do a greater number of justified beliefs indicate greater autonomy?

In Gideon's case, addition of the justified belief that bypass surgery can cause cognitive impairment meant greater autonomy in his choice of treatment. However, endowing him with further information about surgery, even facts of impeccable provenance, seems not to have a similar effect. If

Gideon were informed that bypass grafts are stitched with polypropylene sutures or that the saw used to cut the breastbone has titanium-tipped teeth, it seems implausible that his decision could, as a result, be more autonomous. What properties render some beliefs integral and others superfluous to autonomous decisions?

2.2.2 Materiality and Autonomy: The Account of Faden and Beauchamp

Faden and Beauchamp provide a persuasive account of the belief content that is required for autonomous consent to treatment.[28] They argue that people considering medical treatment must understand information that is *material* to the decision, which they define in the following way:

A material description is or would be viewed by the actor as worthy of consideration in the processes of deliberation about whether to perform a proposed action.[29]

What is material is strongly subjective and is contingent upon the individual's principal interests, goals, and values. Consider, for example, two people who require an ear operation. One is a competitive swimmer with an important meet in two weeks' time, the other a grandmother who detests swimming and hasn't entered a pool in years. To prevent complications, the surgeon forbids water sports for a week following the operation. This information is very likely to be material to the swimmer yet unlikely to be material to the grandmother. Therefore, the consent to surgery of the swimmer, but not the grandmother, will be less autonomous if this point is not understood.

The notion that the individual patient ought to be the final arbiter of materiality is not limited to philosophy circles but has also found favor with the legal community.[30] For example, a landmark decision by the Australian High Court in the case of Rogers v Whitaker defined material information as that which "[t]he medical practitioner is or should reasonably be aware that the particular patient, if warned of...would be likely to attach significance to."[31] In this jurisdiction, failure to disclose material information up to a "particular patient" standard leaves the medical practitioner open to claims of negligence, should an adverse outcome arise that might have been averted were the patient more fully informed.

Faden and Beauchamp consolidate the idea of materiality by drawing a distinction between information that is material to the person deciding and that which is merely *relevant* to a medical procedure. Relevant features are simply those forming part of the object of inquiry. Thus, the timing of an operation, the type of surgical instruments used, and the number of theater nurses involved might all be relevant to a particular surgery.

However, unless the patient deems those facts significant, they are not material to the consent decision.[32] It follows from this approach that if failure to hold a justified belief is to impair autonomous consent, it must relate to a material fact. Belief failures concerning facts that are only relevant do not diminish autonomy. Therefore, if a patient mistakenly believed that silk rather than nylon sutures would be used in surgery, then, given that the type of sutures is immaterial, the misunderstanding does not compromise the autonomy of consent.

Faden and Beauchamp stress that material issues are best discerned through dialogue, rather than a monologue of disclosures by the doctor.

Professionals would do well to end their traditional preoccupation with disclosure and instead ask questions, elicit the concerns and interests of the patient or subject, and establish a climate that encourages the patient or subject to ask questions. This is the most promising course to ensure that the patient or subject will receive information that is personally material—that is, the kind of description that will permit the subject or patient, on the basis of his or her personal values, desires, and beliefs to act with substantial autonomy.[33]

This specification carries strong relevance for elucidating issues of material significance to those with depression through psychotherapy and will be alluded to in more detail in chapter 6.

But does the formulation of Faden and Beauchamp offer a means of quantifying autonomy through an assessment of justified beliefs? From their account we might tentatively suggest that the more *material* facts the agent believes, the greater the autonomy of his or her subsequent, related, decisions and actions. However, before this proposition is embraced with any certainty, some difficulties must first be addressed.

2.2.3 Problems for a Direct Relationship between Justified Beliefs and Autonomy

Reconsider Gideon, who chose medication to control his symptoms of coronary disease. Imagine an alternative scenario where Gideon decides instead to undergo bypass surgery. He consents to surgery with a requisite understanding of material facts but faces an obstacle in the form of extreme needle phobia. In fact, the thought of a needle is so frightening that his resolve to have the operation wavers. Even when the anesthetist assures him that the needle can be inserted after he is drowsy from anesthetic gas, the paralyzing fear persists. After much anguish, Gideon finally hits on a strategy to overcome his phobia: he will be hypnotized to believe that no needle is involved. Hypnosis is successful, and Gideon proceeds to the operation uneventfully. It seems here that *failure* to hold a justified belief about a material fact has facilitated an autonomous decision. Is this a problem for a direct relationship between autonomy and justified beliefs?

A first point to consider is whether the needle is truly material in this case. If it is merely *relevant*, then, on the favored account, Gideon's failure to appreciate the fact of a needle does not impair the autonomy of his consent. However, given that materiality describes features that might impact on a person's interests, Gideon's dramatic aversion to the needle would seem to affirm its material status.

I think a plausible response can still be made to the objection: Gideon's intentional self-deception in fact works *against* his autonomy while at the same time *advancing his interests*. Although diminished autonomy tends to set back interests, and greater autonomy often promotes interests, these relationships are not immune to variance.[34] To illustrate, accept for a moment that Gideon undergoes bypass surgery ignorant of the risk of cognitive impairment. That information is material, and so failure to understand it undermines the autonomy of his consent. However, Gideon happens to be one of the lucky 20 percent who have surgery with no resulting cognitive dysfunction. The result is the best possible in that his writing skills remain intact and he can play tennis and jog without pain. A less-than-autonomous consent has advanced Gideon's overall interests. Similarly, an unjustified belief about a needle anesthetic might impair the autonomy of the original consent while leading to a favorable prudential outcome.

However, the two cases are not parallel. Where Gideon is ignorant of the cognitive side effect of surgery, it seems to be a matter of luck that the outcome favors his overall interests. In the needle phobia scenario, ignorance seems to *reliably* further Gideon's interests. Cases of this second variety, where autonomy is held back yet interests seem predictably advanced, might lead us to wonder where the value of autonomous consent lies.[35] However, it is doubtful, I suggest, that interests are truly served in cases such as this. To see this, it is helpful to shift focus from the preoperative to the postoperative environment. It is very likely that, after surgery, Gideon will chance to see the needle protruding from his arm. In addition, he will face blood tests and additional monitoring needles placed in veins and arteries. It is unlikely that self-deception through hypnosis or any other means will be an effective antidote to his phobia in these circumstances. The fact of a needle is material to autonomous consent, at least in part, because understanding it allows Gideon to prepare effective strategies to lessen his phobic response. Considering surgery in its wider perspective makes it plausible that autonomy promotion aligns more with advancement, rather than hindrance, of interests.

2.2.4 Quantifying Autonomy through Justified Beliefs

The preceding discussion suggests that justified beliefs concerning material facts are necessary for autonomy. The holding of justified beliefs forms a conceptually robust element of autonomy even when broadly conceived across four important contemporary accounts. In addition, it seems fair to assert that the more material facts an agent understands, and believes, the greater the autonomy of that agent's related decisions. To gain understanding of a material fact augments autonomy; to fail to understand a material fact undermines autonomy. In consequence, justified beliefs are a means by which autonomy might be quantified, at least in relation to one of its necessary conditions. This property has value in the clinical context, which will be demonstrated in chapter 4, when autonomy is examined in relation to the person with depression.

At this point it is useful to synthesize the salient elements of autonomy into a working account that will form the basis of the arguments that follow. Autonomy is here conceived as self-direction, encompassing two broad requirements of agency and liberty. Agency implies that power to act, and subsequent control of actions, derives from agents themselves and not from an external source. Desire-based theories of autonomy aim to describe those overarching values and goals that are truly those of the agent and specify that decisions and actions that cohere with deeply held values are emblematic of those under full agential control. Liberty in its negative sense entails freedom from serious impediments to action and in its positive sense mandates the provision of those resources necessary for agents to realize their important projects. Underpinning the formation of values, goals, desires, and their correlative decisions is a sound epistemology based on the holding of justified beliefs about material facts, those facts with a bearing on the agent's pivotal interests. This epistemic foundation is necessary to raise the prospects that actions will ultimately realize aims that are fully those of the agent.

While I have, thus far, tried to convey what autonomy is, it is a very different task to explain why this trait has value. However, if we are to care about promoting autonomy in depression, and if I am to successfully prosecute the case that doctors are morally obliged to do this, it is essential to establish the nature of autonomy's value. A starting point is to examine medical paternalism, which patient autonomy has increasingly displaced as a governing principle in the doctor–patient relationship.

2.3   From Paternalism to Autonomy

Paternalism has cast an enduring shadow in medicine. However, in recent decades its preeminence in the physician–patient relationship has been challenged. In particular, emphasis on the importance of personal autonomy has begun to erode support for paternalistic medical practice. In this section, I look at the reasons behind this transition. An appreciation of why respect for patient autonomy has supplanted long-standing medical paternalism affords insight into the value of personal autonomy and why it ought to be promoted in those experiencing depression.

Paternalism, as its name implies, shares many features with the relationship of parents to their children. Parents usually aim to act in their children's best interests. They do so in the knowledge that children are limited in what they can contribute to an assessment of their own interests. That limitation relates to, among others things, immature rational faculties and lack of life experience. In a similar way, paternalistic medical practice is premised on the assumption that patients lack the capacity to use medical information in a way that will further their interests. Paternalistic physicians utilize this presumption as grounds to withhold medical information, limit discussion of management options, and invoke a demeanor of authority when making treatment recommendations. Pellegrino and Thomasma describe medical paternalism in the following way:

Paternalism centres on the notion that the physician—either by virtue of his or her superior knowledge or by some impediment incidental to the patient's experience of illness—has better insight into the best interests of the patient than does the patient, or that the physician's obligations are such that he is impelled to do what is medically good, even if it is not "good" in terms of the patient's own value system.[36]

Pellegrino and Thomasma point out two principal reasons for the rise of paternalism, or what they term "beneficent authoritarianism," in medicine.[37] First, in past centuries the educational disparity between physician and patient was greater than it is now. As a result, it seems probable that many patients were deemed incapable of comprehending relevant medical information. Perhaps, also, physicians felt free to exert their authority over those who were disempowered by inadequate schooling. Second, the authors point out that physicians were regarded as possessing an almost divine ability to remedy illness, a faculty known, after the ancient Greek god of healing, as "Aesculapian power."

Aesculapian power was a major ingredient of cure. It rested on faith in the quasi-hieratic power and authority of the physician as a person. Indeed, the physician was part and parcel of the cure.[38]

However, in recent years medical paternalism has come under increasing scrutiny. Better education means many patients are now well equipped to assess information about their illness and its possible treatment. Also, the advent of the Internet provides many with rapid access to a wide range of medical data, albeit of varying quality. As a result, people are more able to challenge doctors who might be reluctant to discuss all relevant treatment options or who are less than forthcoming in explaining risks. In addition, the rise of evidence-based medicine has meant that hard data are more readily available on which to base treatment decisions. Outcomes of particular treatments, or of no treatment, can now be framed as probabilities. Although these figures pertain to populations and not to individuals, they are potentially relevant to many choices of medical care. In addition, in some regions practitioner-specific performance data are available to patients.[39] These so-called "report cards" detail the operative outcomes of individual surgeons. While some doctors have expressed concerns that report cards will lead to defensive medical practice and the avoidance of "high-risk" patients,[40] it is likely that many prospective patients would find this information useful.

Given the availability of sound medical information, and the capacity of many people to comprehend it, the withholding of treatment-specific facts is increasingly difficult to justify. A case might give some perspective here. Allen Buchanan describes a malpractice hearing concerning a surgeon who performed a thyroidectomy.[41] The operation resulted in paralysis of the patient's vocal cords, a recognized complication that had not been explained to her prior to surgery. Buchanan quotes the following extract from court records:

The physician was asked, "You didn't inform her of any dangers or risks involved? Is that right?" Over his attorney's objections the physician responded, "Not specifically...I feel that were I to point out all the complications—or even half the complications—many people would refuse to have anything done, and therefore would be much worse off.[42]

The physician appeals to paternalism as a warrant for failing to disclose many potential risks of thyroid surgery. This is evident in his opinion that the patient would be, "worse off" should she forgo surgery. As Buchanan explains, justification for paternalistic practice of this type is grounded in what he terms, "the prevention of harm argument," which can be briefly stated as follows:

1. A physician's primary duty is to prevent or minimize harm to the patient.
2. The provision of certain information will harm the patient.
3. It is therefore permissible to withhold the information in question.[43]

However, the prevention of harm argument is susceptible to criticism on at least two counts. First, it is by no means obvious that a physician is capable of determining, unilaterally, whether provision of particular information would harm the patient in question. To make such a determination seems to entail a value judgment, on the part of the physician, about the nature and degree of any given potential harm. Yet, it is evident that such an assessment goes beyond the purview of the doctor's expertise. Although the physician might be well placed to enumerate, for example, the risks of a contemplated operation, the physician's competence does not extend to determining what value a patient might accord those risks. As Buchanan and Brock have noted,

while the physician commonly brings to the physician–patient encounter medical knowledge, training, and experience that the patient lacks, the patient brings knowledge that the physician lacks: knowledge of his or her particular subjective aims and values that are likely to be affected by whatever decision is made.[44]

Moreover, as Buchanan notes, it does not follow, even granting that the provision of certain information will harm the patient, that it is then permissible to withhold it.[45] For such an argument to hold, it would be necessary to show that the harms of providing such information outweighed the harms of withholding it. It is highly questionable that, in relation to a competent[46] patient, such an assessment could be made without the patient's input. Of course, this means that some patients will receive information that, in hindsight, they might prefer had been kept from them. Nevertheless, as I will argue shortly, such disclosures are warranted because of the value accorded autonomous choice and because of the necessarily subjective element to an assessment of best interests.

Paternalism in medicine is encapsulated by the adage "Doctor knows best." To see why the doctor might not always know what is best for the patient, it is necessary to have some understanding of what have variously been termed theories of prudential value, interests, well-being, or simply the "good." This broad topic will only be given brief treatment here; however, enough will be said to give context to the overall argument.

2.3.1 Theories of Prudential Value

Theories of prudential value generally fall into two categories, subjective and objective. There are two prominent subjective theories. Firstly, mental statist accounts hold that what is good for someone is to achieve a desired experiential state.[47] These accounts include Narrow Hedonism, which measures well-being strictly in terms of the degree of pleasure attained or pain avoided. They also include Preference Hedonism, which holds well-being to align with the mental state that results from satisfaction of the agent's preferences. Preference Hedonism derives from the observation that, to use Parfit's examples, there seems to be a different phenomenal character to the pleasure we feel when listening to music, solving an intellectual problem, or reading a tragedy.[48] On a mental statist account, then, a beneficent medical treatment is one that results in a specified "state of feeling."[49] On the second type of subjective account, desire fulfillment, or preference satisfaction, is held to underpin well-being, independent of the associated mental state.[50] Desire-based accounts hold, therefore, that patients' interests can best be determined by ascertaining their rational and adequately informed preferences. Finally, objectivist accounts, or what have been termed "objective list" or "ideal" theories of interests, hold that certain things just are good or bad for us, whether we desire them or not.[51] For example, love, friendship, health, freedom, and equality of opportunity have all been proposed as universal goods, regardless of individual preference. On an objectivist account, what is good for patients can be determined without reference to their desires, aims, or values.

Medical paternalism, then, in appealing to goods that are independent of the patient's own value systems, appears grounded in an objectivist conception of interests. Thus, the surgeon described in the previous section might attempt to justify withholding information about complications of thyroid surgery on the grounds that the operation was simply good for the patient, irrespective of her own competent views. However, an initial concern with this kind of justification for paternalistic practice is its vulnerability to manipulation by physicians, who might elevate their own values to the ranks of the "objectively good." As Buchanan and Brock put it,

[s]anctioning employment of ideal theories of individual well-being...inevitably invites substantial and unjustified abuse in which others, commonly physicians but also family members, substitute their own conceptions of where the patient's well-being lies for the patient's own conception of his or her well-being.[52]

Of course, were there good reasons to accept an objectivist account, and physicians' recommendations genuinely accorded with it, then paternalistic medical practice might have firmer moral footing. However, as stated earlier in this section, that an agent's good could be discerned without reference to his or her own goals and values seems implausible. Life plans, whether they include ambitions to be a doctor or to run a marathon, are peculiar to the individual. Although it seems likely that certain ideals of the good could be shared, clearly many are not. Moreover, as Buchanan and Brock argue, even objective theories of interests seem to have a subjective component:

Well-being is....substantially subjective on all three theories[53] in the sense that what makes a particular person happy or satisfies his or her preferences depends ultimately on that person's aims, aspirations, and values, and since happiness and/or preference satisfaction is a substantial part of individual well-being on all three theories.[54]

Thus, even if love, friendship and health, for example, could claim the status of objective goods, subjective factors remain integral to how each good translates into individual well-being. Whom we choose to love or befriend and the particular path we take to health remain matters for individual consideration. Even on objective accounts, how each particular good is achieved is highly idiosyncratic. Ultimately, then, appeals to an objective conception of interests lack force as grounds for paternalistic medical practice. There are good reasons for the physician, wishing to act in the patient's interests, to seek guidance from that patient in determining what those interests might be.

2.3.2 Justified Paternalism

Not all medical paternalism, however, represents unjustified interference in the important choices of patients. Someone who lacked the mental capacity to comprehend and weigh pertinent medical information might well be better off were the physician to make a significant medical decision on his or her behalf. Scenarios of this type represent what Joel Feinberg has termed "weak paternalism."[55] Weak paternalism involves intervention to protect another's welfare when that individual is not competent to make the relevant treatment decision. Arguments justifying weak paternalism are often consent based.[56] That is, they hold intervention in such cases to be warranted because consent to it exists, or would exist given certain contingencies. For example, prior consent might be present in the form of an advance directive. Alternatively, evidence might be adduced that a person would have wanted the intervention were he or she competent to consider it, the so-called "substituted judgment" test. An example here would be a previously healthy person, rendered semiconscious from a head injury, who resists surgery for a readily treatable brain hemorrhage. In this case, substituted judgment supports surgical intervention, which would be an example of justified weak paternalism.

"Strong" paternalism, on Feinberg's account, consists in "protecting a person, against his will, from the harmful consequences even of his fully voluntary choices and undertakings."[57] Arguments for the justification of strong paternalism appeal to ideal notions of the good, considered in the preceding section, that are independent of the values of the affected individual.[58] However, as noted, such arguments lack force, and so interventions grounded in paternalism of the strong variety are widely held to be unjustified.

An important point to consider is whether paternalism might be justified in relation to "means," if not "ends." That is, even if we accept that autonomous individuals are best placed to discern those ends that are good for them, ought we also to accept that they are similarly placed to judge the best therapeutic means for achieving those ends? If patients are not in the best position to choose means, is paternalistic practice warranted to make such a judgment for them?

Consider a previously well person who develops appendicitis, desires to return to good health, but refuses appendectomy in favor of treatment with antibiotics. While this course would normally contravene sound surgical guidelines and practice, there are reported cases of success.[59] Here, justified paternalism would require the patient be judged incompetent to refuse treatment, a judgment that would, in turn, hinge on, among others, a finding of irrationality in relation to material facts. For argument's sake, grant that antibiotic treatment is less likely than surgery to produce good health. Incompetence should be deduced if the patient believes antibiotics are *more* likely to be successful. On the best available data, this belief is unjustified and, because it relates to a material fact, it precludes autonomous and competent refusal. Paternalistic intervention might then be warranted, contingent on weighting any liberty deprivation against the degree of expected benefit. However, the situation is different if the patient accepts the evidentially stronger view that antibiotics are less effective yet, because of the value the patient places on, say, avoiding surgery and its potential complications, wishes to pursue this less promising option. In this scenario competence is not impacted upon. Here, the surgeon and patient diverge in the *value* each places on the probability of given outcomes, classed as risks and benefits. A premium placed on a subjective conception of interests mandates deference to the agent's weighting of risks, on the proviso that the quantum of statistical risk itself is accepted. Paternalism is not justified in this situation.

2.4   The Value of Autonomy

That patients with intact decision-making capacity are warranted in refusing interventions that a physician believes to be good for them is grounded in the principle of respect for personal autonomy. The frame shift in medicine away from paternalism and toward autonomy is premised on the value accorded the latter principle. An understanding of the value of autonomy grounds an appreciation of its normative weight and is, therefore, essential for the argument to come. Philosophers generally distinguish between the instrumental and the intrinsic value of autonomy.

2.4.1   Autonomy as Instrumentally Valuable

The account that sees autonomy as instrumentally valuable holds that through autonomous actions agents are best able to fulfill their interests. This account appeals to claims that individuals are, in general, best placed to judge what is good for them, and enhanced autonomy promotes that capacity. Its philosophical underpinnings can be traced to John Stuart Mill, who argued that respect for autonomy has value largely for what it contributes to overall utility. Utility is promoted when individuals pursue their own conception of the good, as long as others are not harmed in the process.

The only freedom which deserves the name, is that of pursuing our own good in our own way, so long as we do not attempt to deprive others of theirs, or impede their efforts to obtain it. Each is the proper guardian of his own health, whether bodily, or mental or spiritual. Mankind are greater gainers by suffering each other to live as seems good to themselves, than by compelling each to live as seems good to the rest.[60]

Transposing this account to the medical model, it seems value might be accorded to respect for the autonomous decisions of patients because, in so doing, their interests are furthered. There is some empirical support for this assertion. For example, the exercise of autonomy, through informed consent, has been shown to contribute to more favorable operative outcomes.[61] This is postulated to result from greater opportunity to develop coping strategies. Thus, being forewarned of a postoperative contingency, such as pain, can lead to preemptive strategies to reduce it. In addition, adequately informed consent can reduce anxiety stemming from ill-founded beliefs about the nature of the operation and its sequelae. Less anxiety generally equates with a lower requirement for anesthetic, sedatives, and pain-killing drugs and, hence, a lower risk of their associated complications. From this, enhanced autonomy can be seen as an instrument to the good of the patient.

There are also prima facie reasons to think that autonomous health care decisions might ultimately lead to outcomes that are in a patient's best interests. To see this, recall the discussion of interests in the previous section. I argued that any plausible account of interests contains a significant subjective element. Therefore, decisions that balance the risks and benefits of a contemplated health care intervention need to take into account the individual's particular goals and values for that individual's interests to be properly served. Further, in order to weigh the relative merits of a certain procedure, the individual needs to be adequately informed and rational. A substantially autonomous individual will demonstrate an adequate understanding of material facts and have a capacity to rationally consider them. Thus, it seems that respecting the patient's autonomy, through ensuring informed consent, leaves the patient well placed to choose in a way that advances his or her significant interests.

Discussion of the instrumental value of autonomy in medicine must make some reference to adverse outcomes of medical research. It is in this domain that some of the most egregious consequences of a failure to respect personal autonomy have occurred. The most heinous example is that of atrocities committed, ostensibly in the name of medical science, by Nazi doctors during the Second World War. In these experiments, subsequently detailed in the Nuremberg trials, the wishes of study subjects were ignored or never sought. Serious injury and death were common outcomes. It is perhaps trivial to state, in cases that were manifestly torture and murder, that if the autonomous wishes of subjects had been respected, these gross harms would not have occurred. However, the extremes of Nazi experimentation place an indelible stamp on respect for autonomy as at least one necessary safeguard to ensure the legitimacy of human research.

Moreover, despite codification of a process to protect the interests of research participants in the Helsinki Declaration of 1964, failure to respect individual autonomy remained widespread in the medical research community.[62] Henry Beecher detailed a litany of cases in a 1966 article in the New England Journal of Medicine.[63] In one study, researchers performed bronchoscopies, where a tube is passed into an air passage of the lung. This is a diagnostic procedure in which samples of lung tissue are collected that can later be assayed for various diseases, such as cancer. However, in these cases, the operator also inserted a needle into a chamber of the heart, a procedure that was experimental, nontherapeutic, and also appeared to have occurred without the patients' informed consent. Such a procedure carries with it a recognized morbidity and mortality, although Beecher did not detail the extent of complications in this study. Again, it is improbable that many or, indeed, any people would subject themselves knowingly and voluntarily to this kind of intervention.

However, it is too simple to say that the doctor who respects the patient's autonomy necessarily brings about outcomes that are in the patient's best interests. Autonomous patients can make choices whose results are ultimately to their detriment. A person can satisfy rigorous standards of informed consent yet still succumb to adverse outcomes of medical treatment. For example, a patient might make a fully informed decision to have keyhole surgery to remove a diseased gall bladder. She might base that decision on the technique's generally more favorable results compared to the traditional "open" approach. However, she could still be subject to complications, such as perforation of the intestine, which are less likely with the traditional surgical technique. In addition, patients sometimes autonomously choose options that they *anticipate* will work against their interests. Consider someone with morbid obesity, who has been unsuccessful in controlling his weight through standard measures. He now faces the choice of gastric banding surgery, which is considered a last resort. Competent to decide, and fully aware of its risks and benefits, he chooses against surgery, knowing that his problem will likely remain, or worsen, as a result. Whatever weighing of values has contributed to the decision, it has taken place as part of an autonomous choice. This type of decision can be likened to that of a smoker who competently decides to continue smoking while, at the same time, acknowledging that her interests would be better served if she desisted.

However, the possibility of a divergence between autonomous choice and interests does not vitiate the instrumental value of autonomy. It is not a requirement that autonomous actions always result in the best prudential outcomes. The account maintains that the autonomous individual is more likely to realize his or her important interests than would be the case if decisions evinced lesser autonomy. Moreover, as stressed earlier, any formulation of autonomy with practical relevance can require only that foreseeable risks be understood; it cannot demand omniscience. The account leaves open the possibility of autonomously chosen harms, but it would be too demanding to hold that for autonomy to have instrumental value its exercise must always fulfill the agent's interests.

2.4.2   Autonomy as Intrinsically Valuable

The second important approach describes the intrinsic value of autonomy. On this account, autonomy is valued in and of itself, not for any benefit that might flow from its application. Robert Young argues, on these lines, that we provide evidence for the intrinsic value of autonomy when we view it as the object of a noninstrumental desire:

Intuitively, an intrinsic good is a good that is not a means to some further good. So, if autonomy is to be thought of as valuable for its own sake this will be because it is not a means to some further good. My suggestion is that it is so in virtue of being the object of a non-instrumental desire.[64]

Young illustrates his argument with an example from the philosopher Richard Brandt:

Consider a child who is swinging, in a rapturous state of enjoyment. We shall probably think that being in this state of mind...is worthwhile for itself alone. To be in a state of rapturous enjoyment of the experience of swinging is for one's state of mind to have an intrinsic property, on account of which the child's experience is desirable. So we shall say the child's experience is of intrinsic worth.[65]

In contrast to the child's "rapturous enjoyment," which is desired intrinsically, Young argues that the desire for water, when thirsty, is largely instrumental. Water is sought not for any intrinsically valuable property but for its effect to slake thirst. Autonomy, Young holds, is akin to the state of mind of the young child swinging. It has intrinsic worth because it is the object of a noninstrumental desire. Jonathan Glover illustrates a similar conception of autonomy by invoking the trivial rules commonly imposed on British housing estates:

On some council estates, there are regulations about the colour people can paint their front door, the kinds of animals they can have or the sort of curtains that are allowed, and these regulations are much resented. And they would probably be resented even if it were agreed that the estate would look much worse without them. Even in small things, people can mind more about expressing themselves than the standard of the result.[66]

In demonstrating that estate residents wish to exercise autonomous choice, while acknowledging that poor overall outcomes will result, the example suggests that autonomy here is desired noninstrumentally. There is a value in choosing that is distinct from the properties of the outcome.

It is likely, too, that there exist situations in health care where the exercise of patient autonomy is accorded intrinsic value. Consider a competent patient who refuses a potentially life-prolonging intervention that the doctor believes has a high chance of success. In this case, the doctor believes medical treatment to be in the patient's best interests. As a result, to be consistent, that doctor ought also to accept that the patient's exercise of autonomous choice, in refusing treatment, will lead to an outcome that is not in the patient's best interests. What, then, might motivate a doctor to respect the patient's decision? It is certainly plausible that a fear of legal repercussions, perhaps charges of medical trespass or battery, might be motivating factors, but it is also possible that many doctors see the patient's exercise of autonomous choice as valuable in itself and base their respect for treatment refusal on an appreciation of that value.

Psychological theories might also inform the question of why autonomy is valued intrinsically. On a prominent view, the prospect of achieving power and control over one's environment forms a central motivation for much human behavior.[67] That motivation is strengthened by the disincentive of power's obverse, namely, defeat, humiliation, and entrapment.[68] It is plausible that individuals derive satisfaction from the exercise of control, and the avoidance of "defeat," in a way that lacks clear connection to the advancement of interests, a claim consistent with the behavior of residents in Glover's housing estate example. Theories of agency, integral to accounts of autonomy, stress a power to act that implies authority not just over oneself but also over one's environment. It is plausible, therefore, that fulfillment of psychological motivations for control might be at least in partial accord with the goals of agency and autonomy and contribute to their intrinsic value. Of course, there may also be "instrumental" goods to which our desire for control permits access. For example, it makes sense that if we cede control to others who may not have our interests at heart, we might be harmed. Nonetheless, this instrumental worth would seem to complement rather than negate the intrinsic value derived from the exercise of control.

Accounts that accord intrinsic value to autonomy are, however, vulnerable to a significant objection. It is plain that dictators, criminals, and the like can perpetrate crimes and inflict suffering through wholly autonomous decisions and actions. Can autonomy retain its intrinsic value if, through its exercise, outcomes result that attract near universal condemnation? To frame the objection in Robert Young's terms, "Is it not the case that the autonomy of the tyrant is the same colour as his (or her) tyranny?"[69]

One response to this type of objection is through noting that autonomy can hold a value that is intrinsic without its being *absolute*. Thus, the value we attach to autonomy, while enduring, must sometimes defer to that of more meritorious goods that warrant greater consideration in a given context. On this basis, we might censure the actions of the autonomous but malevolent dictator through an appeal to the importance of benefi- cence, or perhaps mercy, or forgiveness, without giving up a commitment to autonomy's intrinsic value. However, in resisting the objection, Young adopts a different approach. He holds that the value of autonomy lies in what it tells us of the agent, not in what it contributes to his or her actions. Therefore, for Young, a primary significance of autonomy is its role in our understanding of moral personhood:

The tyrant is so much the worse a person for having autonomously brought about evil. Had he little or no control over his own behaviour he would not be judged so harshly. But if, having the worst of intentions, he sometimes exercises his autonomy ham-fistedly and fails to make life a misery for others, he stands condemned all the same, his failure to bring about harm notwithstanding. Since there is no harm, there is no wrong act. He, however, is not exonerated.[70]

Here, Young concedes that autonomous action can result in serious disvalue. But, he argues, even when autonomous harms are prevented, it is salient that deducing autonomy allows us to assign moral blame to the thwarted evildoer. In that we value the ability to ascribe blame and praise, we ought also, according to Young, to value the autonomy that permits those attributions.

Theories of both the instrumental and the intrinsic value of autonomy face important objections, which I do not intend to further address. However, it is enough to note for my argument that, in medicine, there are good reasons to see autonomy as valuable on both intrinsic and instru- mental counts. But, in order to ground respect for autonomy as the source of moral obligations on physicians, more must be said. To this point, I have outlined what autonomy is and why it holds value, but I have not yet explained what gives it moral status. Specifically, why do the choices of autonomous agents have special moral standing such that we are bound to respect and, in certain circumstances, to promote them?

2.5 The Normative Force of Respect for Autonomy

On one view, autonomy's normative moral force derives from its close connection to agential interests or the "good," detailed earlier. To elucidate this point, it is necessary to briefly sketch some guiding tenets in moral philosophy. It is common in moral theory to distinguish between theories of the good and theories of the right.[71] Theories of the good, outlined in the section on prudential value, aim to determine what is in an agent's interests, or what might contribute to his or her well-being. A case was made that a subjective view of interests ought to be preferred, one that equates advancement of agential interests with satisfaction of the agent's informed and rational preferences. It was further argued that both prima facie and empirical reasons support autonomous choice as an effective means of furthering the agent's interests. Autonomy is thus an instrument to the good of the individual who exercises it. While theories of the good aim to determine the elements of well-being, theories of the right specify what kind of "treatment" that good ought to receive or how we should respond to it. Theories of the right can be broadly classed as consequentialist and nonconsequentialist. Consequentialist accounts hold that the moral rightness of actions can be determined solely by reference to their consequences. For the consequentialist, right action is that which brings about good consequences, and, roughly, the better the consequences, the more ethically defensible the action in question. As a result, consequentialist theories advocate that what is morally right is to promote or maximize the good. Utilitarianism, mentioned earlier, falls into this category in holding that the right course is to maximize utility. The instrumental relationship of autonomy with the good is a reason to accord it significance on a consequentialist account. For the consequentialist, if autonomy promotion will increase the overall amount of well-being, then autonomy promotion is the morally required response.

In contrast, nonconsequentialist theories do not use outcomes as the single measure of moral probity but are more concerned with the agent's actions or intentions. Nonconsequentialist theories propound rules that govern moral behavior, and rule transgression generally marks that behavior as immoral even if favorable consequences ensue. For the nonconsequentialist, the proper mode of dealing with the good is not to promote it but to honor it or permit it to be exemplified in the choices and actions of individuals. On this kind of theory, the right comes before the good, in that the rightness of actions can be ascertained independent of their effects to promote or retard prudential value.[72] To illustrate, if a society were to hold liberty to be a good, for the nonconsequentialist the right course would be to respect the liberty of individuals and to bring about conditions that facilitated such respect. The nonconsequentialist would not countenance deprivation of liberty, even if to do so in just a single case would lead to greater overall liberty. For the consequentialist, by contrast, liberty violation in this circumstance would be morally permissible, or even required.

What is the source of the moral imperative attached to respect for autonomy on the nonconsequentialist account? An important view holds autonomy to be a constitutive trait of persons, and that it is the moral status of persons that grounds an obligation to respect personal autonomy. A foundational interpretation of personhood derives from Immanuel Kant, who held the defining feature of persons to be rationality. For Kant, rationality gives cause to differentiate persons from irrational beings or "things."[73] While persons are, by their nature, ends in themselves, things have only relative value and are permissibly treated as means. Rationality sets humanity apart from less rational beings as deserving of moral respect, exemplified in Kant's Formula of the End in Itself, "Act so as to treat humanity, whether in thine own person or in that of any other, in every case as an end withal, never as a means only."[74] A more recent construal holds personhood to be a property of those sentient beings capable of conceiving of themselves as existing through time.[75] This characteristic is shared by most healthy human beings beyond the age of early childhood and, arguably, by some nonhuman primates. A central feature of persons is the possession of varied and intensely held interests, the most significant of which is generally held to be the interest in continued existence. This interest forms the basis for claims by some that only persons can hold a right to life.[76] This claim is grounded in the notion that to have an interest in life is predicated on the ability to conceptualize one's life and, therefore, the "self as a continuing subject of experiences and other mental states." That personhood indicates the individual to have significant interests underpins the idea that persons are vulnerable to being wronged, in the sense of being harmed by having interests set back or thwarted.[77] It is, on this view, because persons can be wronged that we have reason to accord them moral status and to show them moral respect. Because personhood can apply to young children, it is evident that not all persons are fully autonomous. However, full autonomy, for reasons evident when one considers the requirements of agency and liberty, generally co-occurs with personhood. Respect for autonomy thus derives from a concomitant obligation to respect persons.

Thus far, I have specified an account of autonomy, outlined how it generates value, and proposed reasons for its moral weight. In so doing, I hope to have established a firm basis for setting out the kinds of obligations that physicians bear in relation to patient autonomy. I also hope to have persuaded the reader that autonomy is something that is worth caring about. But in order to complete this task, and cement the relevance of autonomy to the treatment of those with depression, I want now to consider how an understanding of the emotional response might contribute to personal autonomy.

3 Autonomy: The Importance of Justified Beliefs about Affect

In the preceding chapter, I argued that autonomous action requires the agent to hold justified beliefs about material facts, where materiality describes those contingencies likely to have an impact on the agent's important interests. The beliefs examined thus far have pertained to facts about objects that are mostly tangible, and external to the individual, such as suture material and anesthetic needles. However, what of facts about the agent's inner state, such as those concerning his or her psychological make up? Could facts about feelings or "affect" be material to autonomy? In the present chapter, I argue that greater autonomy in dealing with incidents that make us emotional is achieved through understanding the emotional response itself. The grounding claim is that emotional responses help us to identify events that are pertinent to our interests, events whose accurate interpretation is, therefore, material to us. I describe how emotion tends to strengthen the conviction with which related beliefs are held, a characteristic with utility because emotion frequently aids realistic environmental appraisals. However, I show that unjustified beliefs can also be subject to emotional reinforcement with a resulting negative impact on autonomy. In these instances, I suggest affect affords misleading "evidence" for its related cognitions and can be said to have low "evidential value." I invoke theoretical and empirical data showing emotion to be a powerful motivator of behavior and an indispensable element in decision making. These two facets of emotion buttress the chapter's conclusion, that justified beliefs about the evidential value of affect are crucial for the autonomy of the agent's ensuing decisions and actions.

3.1 Affect and Evaluation

My task now is to show emotion to possess evaluative utility. First, I will demonstrate emotion to be a tool that can be used to determine the properties of its triggering events. This claim will later establish the importance, for autonomy, of the agent's discerning when emotion succeeds and when it fails as an evaluative instrument. Second, I show emotions to comprise signs that the outcome of their triggering events carries significance for the agent. This claim supports the materiality of factual information about emotional triggers and, thus, the importance of detecting instances where the evaluative utility of affect is diminished.

While the precise composition of emotion attracts continued debate, most accounts agree on some combination of cognition, feelings or "affect," physiological change, and a resulting behavior that has been influenced by the engendered emotion.[1] Romantic jealousy is a representative example. It typically encompasses presumption of a partner's infidelity, jealous feelings, sometimes flushing or nausea, and often a desire to exact retribution on guilty parties. Many psychologists and philosophers believe emotions can tell us important things about the world, that they are evaluative.[2] This view stems from two observations. First, emotions tend to "fit" specific categories of occurrence. Thus, if one is treated unfairly, one might respond with anger, or if one has committed a wrongdoing and is exposed, one may feel guilt or shame. This suggests that emotions can comprise *evidence* for the existence of their characteristic triggering events. The second observation is that emotional responses are most likely to occur when the individual has a significant interest in the relevant encounter. For example, if I see a neighbor's child being taken to hospital in an ambulance, I might be worried and concerned. However, if I arrive home to find my *own* child has been rushed to hospital, I am more likely to be overcome with fear, anxiety, or panic. In this second sense, emotions can be understood as evidence of the value an outcome holds for the individual.

While more will be said about the specific construal of "evidence" proposed to apply to emotions, some clarifying remarks are in order now. As with epistemic justification, theories of evidence are a major topic of attention in epistemology and will not be dealt with comprehensively. However, a prominent view is that evidence in favor of a proposition is that which raises the probability that it is true. On this view, evidence is a "sign, symptom, or mark" that works to confirm a hypothesis, commonly invoked when ascertaining its truth is otherwise problematic.[3] For example, a broken window and a known felon's fingerprints are evidence of a burglary attributable to that individual. However, if the guilty party is caught red-handed, the truth is accessible in a way that obviates the need for a systematic evaluation of that evidence.

In what follows, I will construe the term "evidence" broadly to include the agent's subjective interpretation of information. Thus, "evidence" will refer primarily to data that raise the probability, for the agent, that a proposition is true. The formulation allows for the possibility that, on more rigorous evaluation, what is initially taken to be evidence does not ultimately support the proposition in question. I suggest that more empirically comprehensive data can inform the *value* of the agent's subjective evidence. In this way, I hold data taken as evidence supporting propositions that are, on independent grounds, likely to be false to have low "evidential value." Conversely, information used to substantiate propositions that can be shown otherwise to be true is held to have high evidential value. Within this framework, I explain how emotion can be adduced as evidence for its associated cognitions while alluding to empirical investigation as a means of verifying or refuting the beliefs to which those cognitions give rise. In support of this conception, I offer the analogy of presentation of evidence in a courtroom, where testimonies and exhibits are subject to scrutiny prior to conclusions on their persuasive merit. Judges and juries are the "triers of facts" charged with determining the proper weight to accord each item of evidence.[4] The evidence of emotion is, I will argue, amenable to comparable examination.

I will show that emotion generally has high evidential value. That is, emotion is a mostly reliable indicator of the presence of its typical trigger, and it is also a consistent sign that the agent places value on the outcome of the triggering event. Yet, I also demonstrate that in predictable instances emotions reinforce cognitions with dubious credibility and thus have low evidential value. In the next chapter I show that affect in depression conforms to this category. Here, I conclude that accurate assessment of the evidential value of affect promotes justified beliefs about the affective trigger and furthers the autonomy of the agent's resulting decisions.

3.1.1 Affect as Evidence for a Characteristic Triggering Event: Judgmentalism

Some philosophers label an evaluative view of emotions "judgmentalism," and others term it "cognitivism." Both terms emphasize the inclusion of a belief as an element of emotion and, in particular, a belief about the presence and significance of a given set of circumstances. Jenefer Robinson explains this approach:

According to [judgmentalism], at the heart of emotion is a cognitive state: an emotion either is or essentially includes a judgment or belief...one thing that judgment theorists tend to agree upon is that the judgments involved in emotion are evaluative judgments about a situation in terms of one's own *wants, wishes, values, interests, and goals.*[5]

In developing a view of emotions that accords, in many ways, with a judgmentalist approach, Ronald De Sousa has described emotions as detectors of *salience* in environmental occurrences, with salience denoting events with the potential to affect the agent's interests:

Emotions are among the mechanisms that control the crucial factor of salience among what would otherwise be an unmanageable plethora of objects of attention, interpretations, and strategies of inference and conduct.[6]

For De Sousa, what is salient derives, in many cases, from an emotional valency that is culturally conferred. For example, in Japan it is impolite to look another person directly in the eye, and to do so is cause for shame. On the contrary, in some Western countries it is a sign of weakness to be *unable* to hold another's gaze. De Sousa argues that we understand what kind of situation calls for a particular emotion through cultural conditioning. He calls the pairings of events with their enculturated emotional responses "paradigm scenarios" and sees them as a basis for each person's emotional lexicon:

We are made familiar with the vocabulary of emotion by association with paradigm scenarios. These are drawn first from our daily life as small children and later reinforced by the stories, art, and culture to which we are exposed. Later still, in literate cultures, they are supplemented and refined by literature. Paradigm scenarios involve two aspects: first, a situation type providing the characteristic *objects* of the specific emotion-type...and second, a set of characteristic or "normal" *responses* to the situation, where normality is first a biological matter and then very quickly becomes a cultural one.[7]

De Sousa's reference to "biology" refers to the view that emotions have evolved because they have adaptive significance. An evolutionary perspective sees emotions emerging through natural selection in virtue of their role as catalysts for survival-oriented behavior. Emerging data suggest that environmental occurrences that provoke emotion are detected and responded to more rapidly.[8] It is also likely that such events are more emphatically committed to memory than those that do not generate emotion.[9] Thus, in our evolutionary past, a fearful response to a dangerous predator promoted rapid avoidance behavior and an imprinting of that encounter in memory. In turn, this primed an enhanced response during future exposures to the same threat. At the other end of the emotional spectrum, feelings of contentment, joy, or love might result from success in the pursuit of food, shelter, or a mate, reinforcing those adaptive behaviors.

That all members of our species would have encountered similar environmental threats and advantages heightens the probability of commonality in our emotional repertoire. As a result, some emotions could be expected to be species-typical, hardwired responses to given stimuli, independent of culture. This was the view of the 19th-century philosopher and psychologist William James, who proposed innate, phylogenetically distinct complexes of events and emotions:

Every living creature is in fact a sort of lock, whose wards and springs pre-suppose special forms of key,—which keys however are not born attached to the locks, but are sure to be found in the world near by as life goes on. And the locks are indifferent to any but their own keys. The egg fails to fascinate the hound, the bird does not fear the precipice, the snake waxes not wroth at his kind, the deer cares nothing for the woman or the human babe.[10]

There now exists some empirical support for a species-typical, biologically encoded element to emotion. Paul Ekman argues that given "elicitors," or stimuli, produce predictable emotional responses.[11] Ekman backs this claim with data showing that the facial expression of particular emotions appears to be stable across cultures. He studied people from isolated ethnic groups and, using pictures, measured their recognition of facial expressions including happiness, fear, disgust, contempt, anger, surprise, and sadness.[12] He found that the various groups came to similar conclusions about the emotion represented in each picture. Ekman uses his findings to argue that some emotions are hardwired means of recognizing environmental events with adaptive significance.

It seems likely that both species-wide and culture-specific expressions of emotion coexist. Although a fear of snakes is relatively stable across cultures, there are many provincial varieties of fear. In Japan, for example, concerns about eye contact, mentioned earlier, have led to the emergence of a debilitating anxiety disorder termed *taijin kyofusho*.[13] The disorder stems from an excessive fear of causing offense through inappropriate gaze. *Taijin kyofusho* is a culture-specific manifestation of an emotion that also has triggers that are shared across cultures.

If affect is evidence for the existence of a characteristic triggering event, cultural variations indicate that context has strong relevance for the nature of that pairing. This observation carries importance for a discussion of depression and, in particular, the role of psychosocial stressors in its etiology, which will be examined in chapters 4 and 6. Although events that represent "loss" are typical triggers in depression, precisely what "loss" consists in can vary according to which contingencies are valued in the individual's culture. For example, humiliation, or "loss of face," although a source of distress for those in Western cultures, carries much greater significance in Japan, where it can cause significant psychological harm.[14]

It is worth considering a study that bears on the contention that affect can afford evidence of its characteristic triggers. Ohman and Soares demonstrated that pictures of snakes could evoke fear in subjects with snake phobia, even when those images were presented subliminally.[15] Thus, anxiety was reliably elicited by a snake image in the absence of any corresponding cognition indicating conscious awareness of it. Subsequent data have described the likely subcortical pathways via which the brain's fear center, the amygdala, is activated in order to mediate this response.[16] Imagine, for a moment, that subjects were informed, after commencement of the study, that their fearful responses were occurring right after subconscious exposure to a snake image and that such exposures would be repeated. Given this additional information, it would be reasonable for subjects to conclude that, during the remainder of the experiment, a feeling of fear comprised good evidence for the proposition "I have been subliminally exposed to an image of a snake." Of course, "evidence" here is contingent upon possession of specific background information. Nonetheless, participants would rely heavily on their affective response to make conclusions about the presence of those pictures. The study lends further support to the view that affect can provide evidence for its typical trigger or, in this case, a representation of it.

3.1.2 Affect as Evidence of Value: The Appraisal Theory of Emotion

It was earlier proposed that affect affords evidence not just of a characteristic triggering event but also of the value its outcome holds for the individual. While grounded in an evolutionary approach, this claim has also been defended in the appraisal theory of emotion, made prominent by psychologist Richard Lazarus. The theory holds that emotions flow from appraisals of states of affairs that involve some form of relationship. It is through relationships, the theory suggests, that we come to have the interests and goals necessary for an emotional response. Lazarus summarizes it this way:

An emotion is always about certain substantive features of the relationship between a person and an environment. Although this relationship can occur with the physical world, most emotions involve two people who are experiencing either a transient or stable interpersonal relationship of significance. What makes the relationship personally significant, and hence worthy of an emotion, is that what happens is relevant to the well-being of one or both parties; in effect, each has personal goals at stake.[17]

Lazarus contends that the presence of personal goals is so important that without them emotion would not be possible:

If there is no goal at stake, and none emerges from the encounter, there is no possibility of an emotion taking place...the minimal cognitive prerequisite for an emotion, any emotion, is that one senses a goal-related stake in the encounter.[18]

By implicating personal goals in emotion causation, Lazarus indicates that the agent must ascribe subjective value to an occurrence if it is to have emotion-generating potential. Appraisal theory thus endorses affect as evidence of the value a triggering event carries for the agent. The theory also refers to the tendency of emotions to "fit" corresponding objects, in a way that parallels De Sousa's paradigm scenarios. Lazarus terms the pairings of emotions with their customary objects "core relational themes." Thus,

anger is the result of a demeaning offence against me and mine, anxiety is facing uncertain, existential threat, sadness is having experienced an irrevocable loss, pride is enhancement of one's ego identity by taking credit for a valued object or achievement, and relief is the change of a negative condition for the better.[19]

There is some empirical data supporting the contention that affect signifies the value an individual places on an event outcome. Hsee and Kunreuther conducted a study in which participants were asked to read the following scenario:

You were in Italy last month. You bought a painting there for $100, and had a local company ship it to your home in the US. When the painting arrived, you found it badly damaged. In order to claim compensation, you must drive a long distance to a branch of the shipping company and show them the damaged painting yourself. If you go there, it is certain that you will get a fixed compensation of $100 – the price you paid for the painting. You won't get more or less than that. If you don't go there, you won't get any compensation.[20]

Researchers imbued half of the subjects with a liking for the painting by asking them to read the following passage, "You liked the now-damaged painting very much and you fell in love with it at first sight. Although you paid only $100, it was worth a lot more to you."[21] The remaining subjects were asked to read a "lower affection" description, "You were not particularly crazy about the now-damaged painting. You paid $100 for it, and that's about how much you think it was worth."[22] Each group was then asked to indicate the maximum number of hours they would drive in order to claim the compensation. They were given eleven choices, ranging from "zero hours" to "ten hours or more." The authors found that participants in the high-affection condition were willing to spend an average of 1.23 more hours driving to collect the $100 compensation than those in the low-affection condition.

The results suggest that the same amount of money had different degrees of appeal in the two conditions. The authors hypothesized that the insurance money had compensation value that was a function of both the monetary worth of the painting and the pain, or negative affect, its loss caused the owner. A positive affective response to the painting and negative affect on its loss were associated with an increase in its perceived value. This study suggests that the individual's affective response could indicate the value, or disvalue, to that individual of an event or outcome. The significance of the evaluative properties of affect for autonomy will be detailed in the last section of this chapter. However, for that project to succeed, the function of emotion to motivate behavior, and its essential role in the decision-making process, must first be detailed.

3.2   Affect and Motivation

3.2.1   Frijda and "Action-Readiness"

It is generally accepted that people strive to act in ways that bring about so-called "positive" emotions such as happiness, joy, and love. They also tend to avoid circumstances that promote more "negative" emotions such as fear, sadness, and shame. In so doing, individuals are driven by their emotions to act in a way that is likely to further their interests. This view is grounded in the idea that good feelings comprise a reward, which reinforces strategies that satisfy interests, and bad feelings are a disincentive to repeat behavior that thwarts interests.

In this vein, the psychologist Nico Frijda sees emotions as both signals of events that are relevant to an agent's "concerns" and as promoters of "action-readiness" in order to deal with those events:[23]

[I]n each emotion-eliciting event some concern can be identified, and it can be argued that detecting concern-relevant events is useful for ensuring satisfaction or protection of these concerns.[24]

Frijda classifies emotional responses in terms of their capacity to motivate behavior aimed at promoting the concerns, or interests, of the agent:

Positive emotions tend to result from achieving...conditions of satisfaction, in which case they signal that activity toward the goal can terminate, consummatory behavior can be initiated, or resources freed for other exploits. "Enjoyment" quite often is the name given to the emotion that follows achievement...similarly, many negative emotions result...from threat or harm to some concern. These negative emotions alert the action system that some action should be undertaken to set things right or prevent unpleasant things from actually occurring.[25]

It seems likely that a key to Frijda's action-readiness component of emotion is physiological change. That is, the body's preparedness for rapid behavioral change is predicated on alterations to, for example, adrenalin levels, muscle tone, and heart rate, changes that are commonly seen in emotion. However, some theorists go further and argue that physiological changes are the *primary mediators* of emotion. These theories emphasize the close bond between affect and action and have strong relevance for my claim that justified beliefs about affect augment the autonomy of the agent's associated actions. If affect is a prime mover of action, it is plausible that affect conveying accurate information assists autonomous action. It is worthwhile, then, to examine accounts linking affect and action in more detail.

3.2.2 William James; Emotion and Physiological Change
William James flagged the importance of a somatic element to emotion when he claimed that physiological change is essential for emotion. James's view is that emotionally competent stimuli[26] in the environment are initially recognized by parts of the brain not involved in conscious processing. That sense perception is then transmitted via the nervous system to various body structures such as the heart, muscles, and other viscera, causing alterations in their functioning. The resulting bodily changes are then relayed back to the brain and apprehended, this time as feelings. He argues that our emotions are the feelings that derive from the brain's perception of changes in the body. On James's theory, any associated cognition is engendered subsequent to this initial physiological process:

Our natural way of thinking about...standard emotions is that the mental perception of some fact excites the mental affection called the emotion, and that this latter state of mind gives rise to the bodily expression. My thesis on the contrary is that the bodily changes follow directly the PERCEPTION of the exciting fact, and that our feeling of the same changes as they occur IS the emotion.[27]

James had little doubt about the content and utility of cognitive appraisals that lacked a bodily, and thus an affective, element. He said that such appraisals would entail only a "cold and neutral state of intellectual perception."[28] He felt that the motivational character of emotions would be stunted or lost in the absence of bodily changes:

Without the bodily states following on the perception, the latter would be purely cognitive in form, pale, colourless, destitute of emotional warmth. We might then see the bear, and judge it best to run, receive the insult and deem it right to strike, but we could not actually *feel* afraid or angry.[29]

In a conclusion that strikes many to this day as counterintuitive, James held that the primacy of altered physiology in the causation of emotion was such that

the more rational statement is that we feel sorry because we cry, angry because we strike, afraid because we tremble, and not that we cry, strike, or tremble, because we are sorry, angry, or fearful, as the case may be.[30]

3.2.3 Damasio and the Somatic Marker Hypothesis

A Jamesian conception of emotion has found recent favor with the influential neurologist Antonio Damasio, who marshals evidence for the primacy of a physiological response in the generation of emotion. For example, relevant nerve pathways between peripheral anatomical structures and the cortex of the brain have been identified. Those structures include viscera such as the intestine, as well as sensors that detect muscle tone, local temperature, chemicals released through tissue damage, pH, carbon dioxide, and oxygen.[31] Neurons that stem from these structures have been found to converge on a part of the brain cortex known as the insula, a region that brain scans increasingly show is active during a person's subjective sensation of emotion.[32]

Damasio has conducted experiments that show changes in physiology tend to precede both feeling states and activity in the insula, as registered on brain scans.[33] He advances what he terms the "somatic marker hypothesis" (SMH), which holds that feelings result from the brain's sensing of the body's "internal milieu." On his account, brain states that co-occur with affective responses are "markers" of the state of the body.[34] Damasio presents a parallel view to James[35] in claiming emotion to be the body's physiological change, which he describes as

a complex collection of chemical and neural responses forming a distinctive pattern. The responses are produced by the normal brain when it detects an emotionally competent stimulus.[36]

Feeling, or affect, is the brain's perception of that bodily state. As he puts it, "feelings bear witness to the state of life deep within."[37]

Damasio's theory provides a persuasive mechanism for the close connection between affective states and action-readiness. On his view, affect is a concomitant of a body that is primed for action. Damasio's work extends the insights of William James and is consistent with the view of Nico Frijda that affect has a strong engagement with action. The etymology of the word "emotion" itself is also consonant with this view. It derives from the Latin *motere*, to move, which, combined with the prefix *e*, means to *move away*.

We have seen that affect can provide evidence of the existence of states of affairs and of their value to the agent. The close link between affect and action heightens the salience of accurate assessments of the evidential value of affect for autonomous action. However, Damasio and colleagues have conducted research that has further implications for the link I aim to establish between affect and autonomy. Damasio's group is now one of a number that has found evidence that affective responses are integral to, and perhaps necessary for, decision making.

3.3   Affect and Decision Making

3.3.1   The Case of Elliot: Absent Feelings, Poor Decisions

It is useful to begin an examination of the link between affect and decision making with a case study, that of Damasio's patient, Elliot.

Elliot was an intelligent young man left unable to work after surgery for a brain tumor, which caused serious personality changes.[38] The changes that made Elliot unemployable had nothing to do with intelligence. His postoperative abilities in memory, perception, language, arithmetic, and new learning were all intact. In addition, he was perfectly capable of discerning the available options in a decision-making process. However, when it came to choosing, Elliot was significantly impaired. He had great difficulty making choices, which almost always turned out for the worse. During his brief period of employment after the operation, he would spend hours reading an interesting dossier while neglecting his primary task of sorting files. He lost all his savings by investing in schemes that, to others, smacked of failure at the outset. Elliot's choices were imprudent and rash.

Neuropsychological tests revealed the problem. Elliot was simply unable to generate feelings in response to stimuli that would normally elicit emotion. Elliot was unmoved by dramatic images of collapsing buildings, fires, and people being seriously injured. He couldn't experience the repertoire of horror, fear, or dismay that most would feel on viewing these scenes. Damasio postulated that the brain region damaged in Elliot's surgery, the ventromedial prefrontal cortex (VMPFC), is responsible for both feeling and deciding and that the two faculties are linked.

The hypothesis is supported by a vignette involving another of Damasio's patients with VMPFC damage. The man was asked to choose one of two available dates for his next appointment. The question set in train a prolonged weighing of the pros and cons of each date. The man considered weather conditions, proximity to other engagements, and, as Damasio recounts, "virtually anything that one could reasonably think about concerning a simple date."[39] The patient was no closer to deciding after half an hour of deliberation. With prompting, he finally agreed to the second date.

The contention emerging from these examples is that people must be able to generate feelings about options in order to decide between them. Feelings weight options with a value that biases the chooser toward those associated with positive affect. Without a mechanism for tagging outcomes with feeling, choice becomes difficult or impossible. While the man making his appointment was able to rationally appraise various dates, without feelings he was unable to place a value on any date and thus couldn't decide. For Elliot, inability to register anxiety led him unwittingly to a dubious business venture and eventual bankruptcy.

3.3.2 The Iowa Gambling Task: Empirical Evidence for Affect-Driven Decisions

Seeking empirical support for this view, Damasio has formally studied decision making in people with strokes affecting the VMPFC. Using the Iowa Gambling Task (IGT), Damasio and colleagues compared the risk-taking behaviors and physiological responses of a group affected by VMPFC strokes with those of healthy controls.[40] In the IGT, participants receive U.S. $2,000 in facsimile bills and are asked to choose cards from four decks with the objective of maximizing monetary return. They are permitted to choose from any deck and to swap between decks as frequently as they wish. Decks C and D are the so-called "good decks." Each card in these decks delivers a $50 win, but every tenth card also carries a $250 penalty. Thus, playing from the good decks eventually produces a $250 gain for every ten cards played. In the "bad" decks, A and B, each card pays $100 but every tenth card carries an additional $1,250 loss. Playing these decks leads, therefore, to a $250 loss for every ten cards played. The primary physiological parameter measured during the IGT is the electrical conductance of the skin. Skin conductance increases with perspiration, indicating activation of the autonomic nervous system, which is responsible for the body's "fight or flight" reflexes.

The healthy group showed increased skin conductance when picking cards from the "bad," or losing, decks, and they chose fewer cards from those decks. Their choices occurred *prior to a conscious awareness* of any strategy to avoid those particular decks; however, they were associated with a "hunch" that the losing decks were in some way disadvantageous. This group did not sustain heavy monetary losses. Conversely, the stroke-affected group failed to develop skin conductance changes in response to the bad decks and also failed to avoid those decks. In addition, this group did not experience a "hunch" that the losing decks were disadvantageous. This group sustained heavy losses.

Damasio argues that these data support a pivotal role for emotions in decision making, along the following lines. The VMPFC compares information about an agent's current circumstance with a database of similar previous encounters. Included in the database is a memory of the emotional response to the relevant encounter.[41] If the current circumstance is sufficiently similar, the comparison yields a match and the same emotion is triggered in the new setting. Damasio proposes that well-recognized neural connections between the insula and the VMPFC mediate these effects.[42] Applying this theory to the IGT, subjects with an intact VMPFC sense, and develop negative affect (the hunch), after picking cards that ultimately deliver losses. Negative affect then mediates an avoidance strategy with respect to the "bad" decks. Subjects with impaired VMPFC function are denied the benefits of this affective input to decision making.

Accepting his conclusions, Damasio's work provides empirical evidence for the importance of affect in decision making. If he is right, and decision making and affect are closely bound, then the importance for autonomy of accurate affect-related cognitions becomes more apparent. However, objections to Damasio's thesis need to be considered.

3.3.3 Damasio's Critics

Tiago Maia and James McClelland present empirical data suggesting participants in the IGT have access to more conscious knowledge of the advantageous strategy than is made out by Damasio's team.[43] They argue that more sensitive data collection in the IGT elucidates more explicit understanding by subjects of the nature of "good" and "bad" decks. They conclude that decision making in the IGT is not necessarily dependent upon emotions signaling the threat of monetary loss prior to conscious and rational appraisal of that threat. Should further data support this position, it poses a challenge to the SMH, the theory grounding Damasio's explanation of findings in the IGT. However, even if the objection is borne out, it does not harm the more general case for emotional involvement in decision making. Maia and McClelland found that decisions in the IGT might have been influenced by conscious assessments of the utility of choosing from particular decks. Their findings do not refute a role for emotional biasing of those decisions.

Indeed, a study by van't Wout and colleagues supports affective influence on decisions made by subjects with conscious knowledge of the strategy under investigation.[44] They measured skin conductance responses in subjects playing the Ultimatum Game, where a "proposer" is given an amount of money that must be divided and shared with a "responder." The proposer can offer any fraction of the money, and the responder is free to reject any offer. If the responder accepts the designated amount, both parties keep the money, but if the responder declines the offer, neither person receives anything. Proposers tend to offer around 50 percent of the total amount, and responders tend to reject anything less than 20 percent of the total amount.

The researchers found that rejected offers were consistently associated with increased skin conductance in responders. The favored explanation is that offers below 20 percent are considered unfair, eliciting skin conductance responses indicative of emotional arousal. Emotions were a concomitant and probable mediator, the authors contend, of decisions to reject unfair offers.

In a wide-ranging review of the SMH, Dunn and colleagues noted that behavior in the IGT could be explained with more parsimony than is offered by Damasio.[45] However, they concluded that

[w]hile the psychological mechanism underpinning the SMH therefore seems to require some revision, the neural substrate that Damasio has proposed has been reasonably well supported by the findings to date. Lesion and neuroimaging studies have found that VMPFC, amygdala, somatosensory cortex, insula and related areas are involved in decision-making processes as suggested in the framework . . . therefore, the SMH seems to have accurately identified some of the brain regions involved in decision-making, emotion, and body-state representation, but exactly how they interact at a psychological level is still somewhat unclear.[46]

The object of explicating Damasio's work in such detail is to convey a sense of the importance of affect in decision making. It seems likely that, even if the mechanisms proposed in the SMH and IGT prove to be inexact, theories that see emotion as integral to decision making will ultimately find further empirical support.

3.3.4 Affect and Evaluative Conditioning

While the neural architecture and pathways linking affect to decision making are yet to be precisely identified, the conceptual soundness of that link is suggested by the fervent economic interest it has generated. Advertisers have long exploited the instinctive connection between emotion and purchase decisions through commercials that engender either immediate or hoped-for future happiness as a result of consumption.[47] Recent research in consumer psychology has sought, with some success, to establish a mechanism through which emotive advertising persuades. The most promising current explanatory theory is termed "evaluative conditioning," which has it roots in classical Pavlovian conditioning.[48] Pavlov's original study involved sounding a bell just prior to feeding a group of dogs. Predictably, the dogs salivated at the food's arrival. With time, however, salivation could be elicited simply by ringing the bell, without a requirement for the presence of food. An initially neutral stimulus, the bell, could become the stimulus for a *conditioned* response, salivation. Evaluative conditioning suggests that advertising can work in a similar way. Pleasing music or images are presented simultaneously with representations of the advertised product, so as to bring about positive affect. With repeated exposure to a commercial, the originally neutral stimulus, for example, a watch of brand x, might evoke the conditioned response of positive affect in the absence of any music or images. In line with evolutionary theory, positive affect is associated with more favorable evaluations of the stimulus as well as tendencies to approach and acquire. Evidence now suggests that favorable attitudes to products can be conditioned[49] and that subsequent buying behavior can be influenced.[50] Given that affect is the likely mediator of these outcomes, it is fair to see the advertising paradigm as a potent depiction of the part affect might play in decision making.

Paul Slovic provides a succinct theoretical label that sums up the role of affect in decisions put forward in this chapter.[51] Slovic proposes the "affect heuristic," which, he argues, operates to expedite adaptive judgment:

The basic tenet…is that images, marked by positive and negative affective feelings, guide judgment and decision making. Specifically, it is proposed that people use an *affect heuristic* to make judgments; that is, representations of objects and events in people's minds are tagged to varying degrees with affect. In the process of making a judgment or decision, people consult or refer to an "affect pool" containing all the positive and negative tags consciously or unconsciously associated with the representations.[52]

The affect heuristic is a helpful sobriquet for a concept whose bearing on autonomy can now be specifically addressed.

3.4   Autonomy and Justified Beliefs about the Evidential Value of Affect

The data presented in this chapter provide support for several contentions. First, affect can comprise evidence for the existence of a particular state of affairs. This claim derives from the observation that affect tends to be paired with a characteristic class of triggering event. Second, affective responses can provide evidence of the degree to which an agent values a particular event or outcome. As Richard Lazarus has argued, if there is no interest or goal at stake in an encounter, the potential for emotion is limited or even absent. Next, emotions are powerful motivators of behavior. That emotions can have accurate evaluative content suggests that their motivating power might often be advantageous. Finally, affect seems closely bound to decision making. Given that affect might provide evidence for the existence of states of affairs, and their value to the individual, it is reasonable to see affect as, in many cases, a useful decision-making heuristic.

I now want to address four remaining tasks in order to link the evaluative properties of affect with autonomy. First, I briefly outline some influential formulations in social psychology that systematize affect as an evaluative tool before elaborating the notion of the evidential value of affect. Second, I describe instances where the evidential value of affect is undermined. Third, I posit means by which the agent might identify these situations. Finally, I argue that recognition of circumstances where affect typically carries low evidential value is a key ability for those seeking greater autonomy. The argument grounds claims in the next chapter that affect in depression commonly has low evidential value, a fact whose understanding is central to the promotion of autonomy in this disorder.

3.4.1   The Evidential Value of Affect

The view that affect could comprise a helpful evaluative tool is gaining prominence in the social psychology literature. For example, Schwarz and Clore have advanced what they term the "affect as information" hypothesis. They contend that, just as the facial expression of emotion conveys to *others* how an individual values an occurrence, feelings communicate that information *internally*, to the individual himself or herself. The authors propose the existence of the "How do I feel about it?" heuristic, where introspective access to feelings guides subsequent judgment and decision making.[53] On this view, agents make stepwise inferences such as, "I feel good about it, so I must like it, and I must like it because it has merit." Contingencies that stimulate positive affect will, therefore, be appraised as worthy of consummatory or acquisitive efforts when the agent consults his or her feelings on the matter.

In a related approach, Pham has characterized the informational content of affect as "the logic of feeling" and describes affect having "ecological validity" as a guide to the nature and value of environmental stimuli:

From a feelings as information perspective . . . a person experiencing a specific affective state tends to draw inferences that are consistent with the essential characteristics of the situations that typically elicit this type of affective state. . . . Affective feelings provide a variety of goal- and task-relevant signals to the individual. A major type of signal is of course a signal of value. What feels good must be good.[54]

Pham summarizes data suggesting that affect valency guides attitude direction while affect intensity influences attitude strength. Thus, positive affect correlates with favorable attitudes, and negative affect engenders unfavorable attitudes, with intensely held affect being associated with greater attitude resilience.

Furthermore, Mayer and colleagues have argued that harnessing emotions to guide adaptive thought and behavior is a skill that ought to be viewed as an intelligence.[55] On their model, emotional intelligence comprises four branches, emotion perception, utilization of emotion to direct thought, emotion understanding, and emotion management. To use their example, consider someone visiting a friend in hospital injured after a car accident. Emotional intelligence entails accurate perception of fear and distress in the patient and family, valid subsequent inferences about their state of well-being, proper understanding of why such feelings arise and how they might alter with time, and the ability to distance oneself from one's own feelings in order to demonstrate empathy and compassion to others.[56] Again, a dominant theme is that emotions convey valid information about one's environment.

It is possible to consolidate these approaches, and the accounts presented earlier, in the evidential terms introduced at the start of this chapter. Recall that evidence is here construed as a mark or signal whose presence raises the probability for the agent that a given proposition is true. It is fair to say that the presence of affect generally raises the probability for the agent that a typical trigger has been causative and that the outcome of the relevant event is one that carries value for that agent. For example, a parent's happiness on seeing her child playing in the water connotes well-being in an object of extreme affection. A student's shame on being caught plagiarizing signals a serious misdemeanor with grave consequences. Fear as a car passes perilously close to the bicycle one is riding presages danger to life and limb, and so on. Affect can, therefore, be adduced as evidence to support assumptions about aspects of related environmental contingencies. In these examples, it is plausible that the occurrence of a specific affective response makes the agent more likely to accord factual status to accompanying beliefs such as "My child is enjoying herself," "My future at this university is under serious threat," or "Without evasive action I am likely to be injured." Not only does affect afford reason, in each case, for the agent to see his or her related beliefs as justified, it is also likely to automatically reinforce the conviction with they are held. As Frijda and Mesquita put it,

[emotional beliefs] are strong beliefs, in the sense of appearing to have a high likelihood of being true, or they are felt to be true, period. During jealousy, one is certain that one's suspicion is justified, and that a given sign implies unfaithfulness. During an angry interchange, there is no doubt about evil intent. When in love, there is no doubt about the deep and intrinsic sweetness and devotion of the loved one.[57]

3.4.2 Affect with Low Evidential Value

Yet it is clear that sole reliance on emotions as a source of action-guiding data can lead the agent astray. The evidence of affect is fallible. Consider the following scenario. Aden notices his girlfriend making eye contact with another man at a party. Within seconds, Aden's pulse begins to race, his face reddens, he feels jealous, and he thinks to himself, "She's going to ditch me." He is struck with a desire to punch the man in question. Here, the combination of affect, cognition, bodily changes, and behavior attests to the presence of jealousy and to its rightful classification as an emotion. In evaluative terms, jealousy provides evidence for a warranting circumstance, namely, that the girlfriend is very attracted to, or wishes to seduce, the other man. Jealousy also corroborates a view that Aden has a strong interest in perpetuating his relationship. That interest might reflect an intense affection for his girlfriend or, perhaps, a heightened vulnerability to loss in the setting of fragile self-esteem. However, the evidence of jealousy for infidelity is defeasible, that is, it can be rebutted by stronger evidence to the contrary. Questioning might reveal that Aden's girlfriend was actually perusing drinks placed next to the man who presents the perceived threat. No doubt Aden would subject this testimony to the rigorous scrutiny advocated by John Benson, but if her version is accurate, jealousy would seem to comprise, at best, misleading evidence of betrayal. It is important to note, however, that the evidence of jealousy for the *value* Aden places on his relationship is less vulnerable to refutation. That such intense emotion could arise in the absence of a significant personal investment is implausible.

Continuing the proposed framework, it is manifest that the evidence afforded by affect can vary in quality. Thus, there will be instances when affect raises the probability that, for the agent, a given proposition is true in the face of compelling data suggesting the opposite. Jealousy reinforces a belief for Aden that his girlfriend intends to be unfaithful, yet this turns out not to be the case. Similar examples come easily to mind. The thirsty desert trekker may feel joy on seeing a lake ahead, yet that joy is misplaced if the water source is only a mirage. The returned soldier with posttraumatic stress who panics on hearing a door slam, and is overwhelmed by thoughts the enemy is at hand, is also misled by the emotional response. Following the terms introduced at the beginning of the chapter, affect in these cases has low evidential value in that it reinforces beliefs not supported after comprehensive empirical inquiry. On this nomenclature, affect with low evidential value has a tendency to promote the holding of unjustified beliefs in relation to its triggering circumstances. Affect with high evidential value has a tendency to promote the holding of justified associated beliefs. A comparison by analogy can be made between this grading of affective evidence and the system employed in biomedical research, where findings are categorized according to the quality of evidence they lend to a hypothesis. For example, high grade, or "level 1," evidence derives from a series of randomized controlled trials, and "level 2" evidence comes from a single randomized controlled trial.[58] Lower grades of evidence come from nonrandomized trials and panel consensus, respectively. Data are viewed with greater or lesser skepticism depending on the grade of evidence that exists to support them. Thus, inferences drawn from, for example, a consensus statement might be applied with caution until further substantiated by a higher grade evidential process. The examples of Aden, the desert trekker, and the returned soldier highlight instances where affect has low evidential value. However, empirical data also illustrate the epistemic uncertainty to which emotional appraisals are prone.

In a foundational study, Schwarz and Clore induced either positive or negative mood in participants by scheduling their involvement on a sunny or a rainy day, respectively.[59] Participants were assessed on their current degree of happiness and their overall life satisfaction. Subjects were significantly more likely to report well-being and life satisfaction if interviewed on the sunny rather than the rainy day. The finding, consistent with the tenets of evaluative conditioning discussed earlier, suggests stimulus appraisals can be influenced by affect that arises incidental to, and not as a result of, the stimulus. Affect is elicited by fine weather, about which positive inferences might be legitimately drawn, yet the affective response is misattributed to other stimuli, the agent's life events. This misattribution cleaves the link between affect and stimulus, calling into question the validity of the affective appraisal. Of further interest, when it was suggested to participants that their evaluations might result from weather-induced mood rather than relating to salient aspects of their life, the negative evaluations of the rainy day participants improved significantly. The authors interpreted this to mean that feelings influenced evaluations only insofar as their source was accepted as reliable. If feelings are felt not to be representative of the target being judged, they are less likely to be utilized as an evaluative tool. This finding suggests agents can scrutinize emotional evidence and use contextual information to determine its value, a facility that I will show to be very relevant to those with depression.

Research on advertising and smoking suggests that evaluative conditioning might also undermine the utility of affective appraisal. It is postulated that commercials and product placement in films encourage a view of smoking as the pursuit of the powerful, attractive, and glamorous. This, in turn, is proposed to induce positive affect and favorable attitudes in viewers who value these traits.[60] Positive affect toward an object may lower perceptions of its risks, a finding that is suggested to increase cigarette smoking, against the now very clear dangers.[61,62] A survey of young smokers provides evidence that initially favorable evaluations of smoking, and their probable affective mediation, were ultimately misleading. Eighty percent of respondents answered "No" to the question, "If you had to do it all over again, would you start smoking?"[63] If, by premeditated design, affect and favorable attitude are conditioned toward a product for which we would otherwise hold no special feelings, then reliance on affect to assess value would seem misguided.

These data raise an obvious concern. If affect can possess low evidential value, can it also retain evaluative utility, and if so, how? I want to suggest that affect does retain evaluative utility, and I offer three mechanisms for how this might be so. First, I suggest a reasonable conjecture is that, in psychologically healthy individuals, affect with low evidential value occurs infrequently. By and large, when we feel happy, it is because good things have happened, and if we are fearful or sad, there is legitimate cause to impute threat or disappointment. If one considers the gamut of emotions that are experienced in the course of a typical day, it is, I suggest, unusual to look back and see more than the occasional emotion as misplaced or unwarranted.

Second, there is a plausible evolutionary hypothesis as to why affect with poor evidential value might arise at times yet still carry utility in the form of adaptive advantage. Imagine walking through uncut grass and encountering a thin, coiled, cylindrical object. Your hardwiring primes you to feel afraid, a feeling that encourages certainty in your belief that the object is a snake, and a desire to run. Yet the object may well be a garden hose, and that could be ascertained through brief inspection. On an evolutionary explanation, fear primes us to believe the worst-case scenario as part of a "better safe than sorry" strategy, which limits the *cost* of mistaken identity, without necessarily limiting the *number* of overall mistakes.[64] Thus, while a single failure to take the object to be a snake could be fatal, many failures to take it to be a hose could occur without serious consequence. In short, there is an adaptive function in holding affect-associated cognitions to be true, whose corollary is that affect will sometimes sustain cognitive errors. This kind of theory also explains why people have difficulty relinquishing affective beliefs, even when sound data contradict them. Fear of flying is a classic example of affect's persisting against the dictates of reason. This point will gain relevance in chapter 4 when the impelling nature of depressed cognitions is discussed.

Finally, and perhaps of most relevance for the autonomy argument here, humans have a unique capacity for reflective self-evaluation. This implies an ability to discern those emotional beliefs that are confounding from those that are validly action guiding. The individual who is alert to the possibility of affect with low evidential value is well positioned to be cautious in utilizing his or her affective response as a basis for decision making. This kind of self-awareness requires agents to possess two key abilities. They must be able to determine the evidential value of their own affective responses and also to recognize circumstances when such a determination is indicated. I want now to posit means by which these goals might be achieved.

3.4.3   Determination of the Evidential Value of Affect

Paul Slovic has suggested the affective input to decision making be construed as a heuristic. Accepting this account, a technique for measuring the evidential value of affect might be gleaned by examining the function of heuristics more generally. Heuristics are "mental shortcuts" brought to bear as a means of simplifying decision making under uncertainty when appraisal of relevant data is complex and cognitively demanding. For example, the distance of an object can generally be ascertained by its clarity.[65] More distinct objects are usually closer than those that are less well-defined. However, distance can also be calculated by more laborious methods, such as measuring the number of paces between target and observer. While this heuristic is mostly reliable, it is prone to biases that are often systematic and predictable. For example, in the presence of fog, proximate objects appear indistinct and might be mistakenly believed to be distant. It makes sense that in foggy conditions the informed observer would exercise caution in relying on the visual cue of distinctness as a means of assessing distance. If the pacing method is feasible, then it appears to offer a more consistent measure that is less vulnerable to variance as a result of biasing effects. In a similar way, if there were concerns about biased affect, assumptions generated as part of the affective response could be subjected to empirical scrutiny. For example, the happy poolside parent could verify positive affect as a legitimate indicator of his or her child's contentment through simple inquiry or by moving closer to seek visual or auditory cues. The shameful student could elucidate the predictive validity of his or her negative affect by meeting with teachers for precise information about the repercussions of plagiarism for his or her academic future, and so on. Thus, it is plausible that, if alternative sources of information about the target object are available, and the agent is able to commit resources to their exploration, this kind of empirical investigation affords the clearest means of fully evaluating the significance of an affective stimulus.

Whereas fog would seem to reliably confound assessments of distance, the existence of any similar indicator of biased affect remains to be shown. Might there be predictable circumstances under which the affect heuristic yields inaccurate ecological data and thus presents as a specious guide to action? Awareness of such circumstances could alert the individual that the emotive target warrants more methodical analysis before action is taken.

A starting point is to isolate instances where the affect heuristic is most likely to be engaged as a decision tool. It is plausible that when affect is relied upon at the expense of a more systematic evaluation of data, there is greater opportunity for misleading affect to drive action. On one account, we are more likely to be guided by the heuristic value of affect, and less likely to question its related evaluations, when other avenues of explanation are relatively inaccessible. As a result, we are more likely to rely on heuristics in situations of time pressure, or when under "cognitive load," that is, engaged in tasks that make additional demands on our cognitive capacities.[66] A suggestion, then, is that the agent be alert to the possibility of affective biases under these conditions and be prepared to commit to fuller evaluations wherever possible.

A further pertinent line of research suggests specific emotional states can be accompanied by appraisals that are held with greater or lesser certainty. For example, individuals experiencing anger and disgust display relative confidence that they understand a situation and can predict its outcomes. Conversely, fear, surprise, and worry are associated with greater uncertainty as to the nature of a target state of affairs and its likely sequelae.[67] Further, there is evidence that appraisals that are held with certainty are more likely to be prone to heuristic rather than "systematic" processing, a dichotomy recognized in "dual process" theories of cognition. Heuristic processes are "spontaneous, quick...and reliant on rules of thumb," whereas systematic processes are "thorough, detailed, careful, and reliant on analysis."[68] In a study demonstrating this effect, participants were induced to experience either a "certain" emotion such as anger or an "uncertain" emotion such as worry.[69] They were then asked to read an article whose author argued that grade inflation was a big problem in universities and that students should be marked more severely. Some read the article framed as a newspaper editorial written by a distinguished professor, while others read the identical article presented as a college student paper. Those experiencing "certain" emotions were more persuaded on reading the expert as opposed to the nonexpert source, whereas those experiencing the "uncertain" emotions were equally persuaded by both articles. The finding suggests the "certain emotion" condition promoted reliance on the heuristic cue of "expert authorship," whereas the "uncertain emotion" condition facilitated a more "systematic" evaluation of the argument. While it can only be conjecture at this point, perhaps emotions such as jealousy and anger, which seem to engender great conviction in the beliefs they generate, are associated with greater reliance on the affect heuristic and a lower propensity to systematically evaluate triggers. If so, it is plausible that actions arising from "certain" emotions might be more vulnerable to unreliable affect and less fully informed than those based on their "uncertain" counterparts. Agents might then be cautioned to be circumspect about the credibility of assumptions made under these conditions.

I want to further suggest that our intuitions about an emotion's track record of action-guiding utility might also be helpful. For example, jealousy and anger present as two emotions that seem to correlate with hasty actions leading to consequences that are later regretted. Perhaps on this basis we might say that those experiencing such emotions should be alert to their history of poor evaluative reliability, or low evidential value. There should, therefore, be a correspondingly greater effort made to empirically verify the kinds of cognitions that drive behavior in such cases.

However, there is a final class of affect where evidential value is routinely poor. Affect arising in psychological disorder promotes the holding of false beliefs to a much greater extent than does affect in the healthy individual. Here, affect frequently comprises a low grade of supporting evidence for related cognitions. It is my goal in the next chapter to show that the evidence afforded by affect in depression fits this category and that the autonomy of the depressed person is greatly dependent on understanding this fact and appropriately responding to it. To ground that argument, however, it is necessary to detail the link between agents' understanding of the evidential value of their affective response and the autonomy of their resulting decisions and actions.

3.4.4   Autonomy and the Evidential Value of Affect

In the previous chapter, I argued that personal autonomy is predicated on the agent's holding justified beliefs about material facts. Invoking the account of Faden and Beauchamp, material information was defined largely in subjective terms, as that with the potential to impact on the individual's important *values, goals, and interests.* It is timely, then, to recall that affect tends to arise when the individual's important goals and interests are at stake. This is central to the appraisal theory of Richard Lazarus and is consistent with the view of Nico Frijda, who sees emotions as signals that action is required to protect the agent's "concerns." These observations lead to a claim central to the present argument; *affect-associated cognitions pertain to aspects of the affective trigger whose factual basis is likely to be material to the agent.* Consider again the case of jealous Aden. Whether his girlfriend is contemplating the drinks counter or another man is highly pertinent to his interests and is likely to be material to him. Moreover, his affect-associated cognitions are likely to relate to that material information, for example, "My girlfriend is looking at another man. She wants to leave me." The presence of jealousy indicates the truth of its related cognitions to be a material matter for Aden. Further parallels with the account of Faden and Beauchamp can be drawn to clarify the position I take here.

It is unlikely that Aden's affective beliefs will pertain to, for example, the color of his girlfriend's dress, or what she is drinking. These aspects do not bear on his significant interests and hence do not contribute to the generation of affect. These facts might thus be classed as "relevant" to the object of the emotion, but not material to Aden's consequent decisions.

Accepting the argument thus far, it follows that an understanding of the factual basis of affect-driven cognitions is important for the autonomy with which an agent decides and acts in relation to the affective trigger. Autonomy, it will be recalled, requires a sound epistemology where material matters are concerned so that decisions and actions will have the greatest chance of reflecting the agent's important values, satisfying those goals that are of greatest priority, and exerting effective control in the relevant circumstance. Whether Aden decides to confront his girlfriend, accost the other male, leave the party, cast doubt on the future of the relationship, or none of these, hinges in large part on the credibility he accords his jealous assumptions. Correctly designating those assumptions justified or unjustified advances the autonomy of his final decision, permitting him greater control over relevant outcomes and heightening the chances that his salient interests will be furthered. This effect is emphasized when one considers the close relationship between affect and both decision making and action, considered in the preceding sections. If the favored accounts are accepted, affect will exert a profound influence on Aden's ultimate decision. Also, because affect is such a powerful motivator, affect-associated cognitions are very likely to influence his subsequent actions. This is in contradistinction to cognitions that arise without accompanying affect. The significance for autonomy, then, of agents arriving at an accurate evaluation of their affect-driven cognitions, becomes evident.

The preceding discussion supports an understanding of the evidential value of the affective response as central to this goal. If agents are aware that extant affect is of a class likely to reinforce unjustified beliefs about material matters, they are in a better position to subject those beliefs to appropriate interrogation than if they were ignorant of this information. It is an understanding of which affective responses *tend* to have poor evidential value that is pertinent, I contend, to the issue of when to investigate their associated cognitions. Jealousy has been proposed as an emotion with a tendency to give rise to, and reinforce, false cognitions. Alertness to the poor evidential value of this category of affect can lead to a stance of detachment from its related beliefs and assist their empirical investigation. For example, if Aden is aware that jealousy commonly engenders false beliefs, he is better placed to treat those beliefs with skepticism and to test them before acting. In this way, his subsequent actions will be more firmly grounded in facts and will be more autonomous. It is conducive to his autonomy that Aden possesses justified beliefs about the evidential value of his affective response. The caveat is that the existence of distinct sets of emotions with poor evaluative utility remains speculative while relevant research in social psychology is at an early stage. However, I want to show now that much greater confidence is warranted that affect in depression has low evidential value. In the next chapter, not only will I argue this to be so, I will also demonstrate that depressed persons often fail to identify their depressed cognitions as having dubious credibility. When the depressed person says, "I *feel* so bad, my pessimistic thoughts *must* be true," I suggest that "feeling bad" is, in most cases, accorded greater evidential weight than it deserves. Failure to hold justified beliefs about the poor evidential value of affect in depression, I will argue, undermines the autonomy of the depressed person. This claim will form the basis for a comparison of the respective effects on autonomy in depression of CBT and ADM, the subject of chapters 5 and 6.

4 Depression: Disorder of Affect, Disorder of Autonomy

My task now is to show that depression undermines personal autonomy. Such a claim is hardly controversial, as most accept that the depressed worldview frequently misrepresents reality and, on just about any account, sets back autonomy. However, I want to be quite specific about the nature and mechanism of skewed perception in depression, in order to later tease apart the differential effects of psychotherapy and ADM on autonomy in this disorder. First, I will detail the negative information-processing biases that lead to false pessimism and show how depressed affect is a pivotal mediator of this distorted thinking. While acknowledging negative biases as a primary threat to autonomy, I go on to argue that a failure to *understand depressed affect* as a reinforcer of confounding pessimistic beliefs further sets back autonomy. Next, I show how stressors can precipitate depressive episodes and that information linking stressful life events to depression is likely to be material to the afflicted person. Yet, I argue that two factors conspire to obscure that connection. First, I show that a prevalent medical conception of depression as a primary disorder of brain chemistry deters the elucidation and management of stressors. Second, I show that negative attributions warp stressor appraisals by overemphasizing personal inadequacies as causal and fostering inaccurate forecasts of wide-ranging and enduring adversity. I conclude that a failure to hold justified beliefs about the poor evidential value of depressed affect erodes autonomy in depression and, more specifically, undermines the autonomy of stressor-related decisions.

4.1 The Cognitive Approach to Depression

I will make claims about biased thinking and stressors in the context of a cognitive approach to depression. It is necessary, then, to provide background on depression generally and on a cognitive theory in particular.

A definition with broad currency comes from the *Diagnostic and Statistical Manual of Mental Disorders*, fourth edition (*DSM-IV-TR*), of the American Psychiatric Association. It states the following:

The essential feature of a Major Depressive Episode is a period of at least 2 weeks during which there is either depressed mood or the loss of interest or pleasure in nearly all activities. In children and adolescents the mood may be irritable rather than sad. The individual must also experience at least four additional symptoms drawn from a list that includes changes in appetite or weight, sleep, and psychomotor activity; decreased energy; feelings of worthlessness or guilt; difficulty thinking, concentrating or making decisions; or recurrent thoughts of death or suicidal ideation, plans, or attempts. . . . The episode must be accompanied by clinically significant distress or impairment in social, occupational, or other important areas of functioning. For some individuals with milder episodes, functioning may appear to be normal, but requires markedly increased effort.[1]

The *DSM-IV-TR* includes an additional group of specifiers of severity. In mild depression, "few, if any, symptoms in excess of those required to make the diagnosis are present, and symptoms result in no more than minor impairment in social or occupational functioning." In depression of moderate severity, "symptoms or functional impairment between mild and severe are present." In severe cases, "many symptoms in excess of those required to make the diagnosis, or several symptoms that are particularly severe, are present, or the symptoms result in marked impairment in social or occupational functioning."[2]

While the *DSM* criteria for depression are an accepted benchmark for most health professionals working in the field, their propagation has also generated controversy. A notable recent critique comes from Allan Horwitz and Jerome Wakefield, who argue that *DSM* improperly merges normal experiences of sadness with diagnoses of depressive disorder. Key to their concern is what they see as the inability of *DSM* to differentiate between sadness as a response to loss or other distressing circumstances and so-called sadness "without cause."[3] On their account, this distinction is crucial, as it is only sadness, or depression, "without cause" that truly qualifies as a disorder.

The contextual nature of much depression is central to my own argument, and I will spend some time elaborating it. And Horwitz and Wakefield might ultimately be shown correct that *DSM* "overpathologizes" many people with quite legitimate sadness in the face of adversity. However, the debate over precisely where to establish the definitional boundary for depressive disorder has only tangential relevance to the claims made here. For my argument, *DSM* criteria are helpful in establishing uniformity between instances labeled as depression and acting as a yardstick demonstrating the comparable efficacy of ADM and psychotherapy. Were the diagnostic criteria of depression to shift, the importance for autonomy of understanding affective biases and the contextual nature of stressor-related depression would, on my account, remain. For this reason, I do not intend to further consider critiques of the *DSM* classification of major depressive disorder.

The cognitive theory of depression, developed by Aaron Beck, has found wide favor with psychological health professionals.[4,5] The psychotherapy based on it, cognitive behavior therapy (CBT), has been shown to be efficacious in extensive clinical trials.[6,7] Although there are many different psychotherapeutic approaches to the treatment of depression, CBT has been the most rigorously evaluated, and its efficacy in depression is the most clearly substantiated.[8] A central tenet of the cognitive theory is that affect and cognition have a mutually reinforcing relationship that contributes to the evolution and maintenance of depressive symptoms. Pessimistic or negative cognitions can trigger and perpetuate negative affect, and negative affect can lead to a tendency to focus and ruminate on negative cognitions. The depressed person sees desired events as unlikely to happen, an inclination termed "hopelessness" in the depression literature. As depression becomes more marked, pessimistic predictions become more pronounced. In severe cases, the depressed person can become *convinced* that feared events will occur. Susan Andersen and colleagues describe the process:

[H]opelessness is best conceptualized as the point at which an individual begins to experience and treat dreaded events (or a single dreaded event) as inevitable rather than simply likely. When dreaded events seem certain to occur they are treated as if they have already occurred and are given a reality that is functionally equivalent to their having already transpired. One is certain enough that one ceases to expend effort; one gives up . . . in this sense hopelessness is best conceptualized as depressive predictive certainty, the point at which dreaded future events are treated as certain to occur or that desired future events are treated as certain not to occur.[9]

Andersen's description alludes to a second defining feature of depression, a sense of helplessness, or inability to alter the unfolding of events. Helplessness is predicated on a broadly negative self-view encompassing inadequacy, worthlessness, and undesirability.[10] A central precept of cognitive theory is that such evaluations are almost always misconceived, or "distorted." The cognitive therapist challenges negative cognitions by inviting the individual to justify them. In many cases negative assessments cannot be substantiated, and it is concluded that, on available facts, more favorable outcomes are likely. The behavioral component of CBT asks the depressed person to pointedly pursue activities that might otherwise be avoided. The therapist highlights any resulting positive experience as further evidence for the falsity of negative predictions. More positive cognitions contribute to the lifting of negative affect and improvement in depression.[11]

That negative cognitions in depression are frequently erroneous is a central contention in the argument presented here. I intend to show that a failure to identify and to correct for unjustified pessimism presents a grave threat to the personal autonomy of those with depression. It is worthwhile, therefore, to consider in some detail the empirical basis for this claim. Are negative predictions in depression really unjustified, and, if so, how do they come about?

4.2   Information-Processing Biases in Depression

4.2.1   Mood-Congruent Processing Biases

A considerable body of evidence suggests a preferential processing of *mood-congruent* information occurs in depression.[12,13] Mood-congruency accounts propose that, in depression, there is greater attention to, and easier recall of information with negative affective content. A corollary of easier access to negatively toned material is an increased frequency of negative cognitions and the subsequent reinforcement of negative mood.

"Attentional" biases in depression have been demonstrated with the dot probe task, which requires subjects to identify the presence of a gray dot on a screen shortly after a parcel of information has been presented. Longer latencies in identifying the dot are associated with increased attention to, and engagement with, the preceding stimulus. Depressed subjects have been found to display heightened attention to and engagement with both negative words[14] and sad faces[15] presented on a screen in dot probe studies. Most work, however, has been done on mood-congruent memory biases in depression, which a number of investigators believe are well explained by a heuristic known as availability.

4.2.2   The Availability Heuristic

Heuristics, alluded to in the previous chapter, are "mental shortcuts," which can assist decision making under conditions of uncertainty. First proposed by Amos Tversky and Daniel Kahneman, the availability heuristic refers to the thought processes that might underpin judgments about frequency and probability.[16] They describe it in the following way:

There are situations in which people assess the frequency of a class or the probability of an event by the ease with which instances or occurrences can be brought to mind. For example, one may assess the risk of heart attack among middle-aged people by recalling such occurrences among one's acquaintances. . . . This judgmental heuristic is called availability.[17]

To use the authors' example, availability suggests that if heart attacks are easier to recall in middle-aged friends than in any other age group, heart attacks will be deemed more common in middle-aged people generally. While Tversky and Kahneman consider the availability heuristic to be an effective guide, they also note that it is fallible:

Availability is a useful clue for assessing frequency or probability, because instances of large classes are usually recalled better and faster than instances of less frequent classes. However, availability is affected by factors other than frequency and probability. Consequently, the reliance on availability leads to predictable biases.[18]

According to Tversky and Kahneman, availability is prone to biases in the "retrievability of instances":

When the size of a class is judged by the availability of its instances, a class whose instances are easily retrieved will appear more numerous than a class of equal frequency whose instances are less retrievable.[19]

This type of bias can favor the retrieval of instances in memory that are, for example, particularly salient. Salience biases are tendencies to overestimate the likelihood that a graphic or extreme experience will recur. For example, a person who experienced terror while catching a burglar red-handed might overestimate his or her chances of being robbed again, compared to someone who was burgled without confronting the intruder. Retrievability of instances is also affected by biases in "cognitive structure," which occur when information is processed according to the individual's specific mental schema.[20] "Schema" refers to an ingrained way of interpreting the world stemming from a person's unique set of experiences. Consider an elderly man who has been hospitalized many times in his small rural town, where the nurses are mostly female and the few doctors are male. After developing an illness requiring specialized care, he is transferred to a metropolitan hospital where roughly half the doctors are female, an accurate reflection of the gender distribution among physicians. On arrival, the man is attended by a female doctor, whom he mistakes for a nurse. If availability is accepted, the mistake relates to a retrieval of instances that is biased by an unrepresentative personal schema. The man holds a stronger association between the female sex and nurses rather than doctors. This leads to easier retrieval of that pairing, and subsequent inferences about the prevalence of female doctors that are at odds with true frequencies across the wider population.

Emerging data now implicate biases in availability as an explanation for the kinds of cognitions that occur in depression. It is likely that those with depressed mood have relatively easy recall of "negative" events, like a relationship breakup or job loss. In contrast, positive events, such as a promotion at work or receiving a compliment, are less readily brought to mind. A study by MacLeod and Campbell supports a causal role for availability biases in depression.[21] They triggered happy and sad moods in research subjects through the use of mood induction statements. This method requires subjects to reflect on propositions designed to bring about specific feeling states. Statements aimed at evoking a positive mood included "I have good friends who really care about me" and "I have so much confidence in myself—I can do anything if I try." Examples of "negative" statements were "I'm so hopeless I'll never be a success" and "Everything I do turns out wrong—I'm incapable of doing anything well."[22] To determine whether induction had been successful, subjects rated their mood on a visual analog scale.

Participants were then asked to recall positive and negative events and to predict the chances of those events' being repeated. "Positive" events included "a successful relationship," "a wonderful holiday," and "a rewarding job." "Negative" events included "a damaged possession," "a sleepless night," and "a frightening assault." Happy mood induction correlated with an easier recall of positive events. Subjects in a happy mood were also more likely to predict that positive events would occur in future. Sad mood induction resulted in easier recall of negative events, and sad subjects thought negative events were more likely to recur. The researchers concluded that good reason existed to see mood-congruent availability biases as the underlying mechanism:

These findings are fully consistent with Tversky and Kahneman's proposal that, when people judge the future likelihood of events, they are indeed influenced by the degree to which past occurrences of similar events can be accessed in memory.[23]

In a slightly varied approach, MacLeod and colleagues wondered whether pessimism in depression might depend on the ease of availability of *explanations* for negative outcomes.[24] The researchers were investigating what role the "simulation heuristic" might play in the neuropsychological mechanism underpinning depression. Kahneman and Tversky have proposed the simulation heuristic to be an extension of their concept of availability.[25] It suggests that people base probability assessments on the ease with which they can mentally simulate a contemplated event or outcome. Thus, the more readily an individual envisages an outcome, the higher he or she will rate its chances of occurring. MacLeod and colleagues posited that depressed people are more pessimistic because they are better able to explain, and thus mentally simulate, negative outcomes.

The researchers asked depressed patients to rate the likelihood of various positive and negative events' occurring and to explain why such events would or would not happen to them. Positive events included "You will achieve the things you set out to do," "You will have good times with friends," and "Your health and fitness will improve." Negative events included "You will have financial difficulties," "You will be unable to cope with your responsibilities," "You will make a fool of yourself in public," and "You will become seriously ill." The investigators found that, compared to a control group without depression, the depressed group judged the negative events to be more likely and the positive events to be less likely. The depressed group was also more able to give explanations for the negative occurrences. Supporting a role for the simulation heuristic in depressive pessimism, the authors concluded their findings were consistent with a "causal link between explanation accessibility and subjective probability."[26] Vaughn and Weary have reported similar findings, showing that depressed mood and easy access to reasons for negative events positively correlates with predictions that such events will occur.[27] Recent reviews suggest the conclusions made in the preceding studies are robust and that they form the basis for plausible assumptions about how negative predictions in depression arise.[28,29]

Mood congruency, encompassing attentional biases, availability, and simulation, is a useful way of conceptualizing the negative information-processing biases that typify depressed thinking. The data presented indicate that depressed people attend more closely to negative information and accord it greater weight when determining the likelihood of future events. The findings also suggest that negative mood promotes preferential access to negative memories as well as to explanations for negative outcomes. These biases are proposed as a mechanism for the tendency of depressed people to make pessimistic predictions. However, the claim that negative biases are active in depression faces an important objection.

4.2.3   Depressive Realism

Proponents of *depressive realism* argue that the predictions of those with depression, rather than being negatively biased, are in fact more accurate than those made by people without depression. On this account, the depressed are "sadder but wiser" and it is the nondepressed who exhibit biased thinking and are irrationally optimistic.[30] Depressive realism has some intuitive appeal. People with depression can generate their own misfortune, with low spirits and irritability sometimes alienating others and fostering poor outcomes. Such outcomes are termed "dependent events" in the psychology literature because the agent's own actions contribute to them.[31] "Independent" events, on the other hand, are unwanted outcomes thought to be outside of the individual's sphere of influence. It is plausible that a person with depression might accurately predict "dependent" negative outcomes—those that his or her own behavior made more likely. For example, if the person believed no friends would call that day, knowledge that his or her own demeanor discouraged friendly overtures could heighten the likelihood of an accurate assessment. It is also reasonable that depression triggered by an unpleasant or stressful event could signify taxing times ahead. In this case, pessimism could be justified in the circumstances and realistically reflect likely outcomes. Moreover, it is probable that people with an especially sanguine outlook could at times evince unrealistic optimism. Misplaced enthusiasm has driven many projects that later failed.

There is also empirical evidence for depressive realism. Those with depression perform better on so-called "contingency judgment tasks," which require participants to predict whether a light will appear when they press a button, but where the experimenter actually controls the light illumination rate.[32] Those without depression tend to overestimate the likelihood that their actions will illuminate the light, a finding termed "the illusion of control." Conversely, the depressed display no such bias, challenging the thesis that pessimism in depression is unrealistic.

However, depressive realism faces a number of difficulties. First, there are conceptual objections for which depressive realism fails to account. Many negative forecasts made by those with depression pertain to events that are not conceivably "dependent." For example, depressed individuals have been shown to predict a greater likelihood of experiencing the sudden onset of serious illness,[33] or of being physically attacked.[34] It is implausible that depressed predictions would be more accurate when they concern events whose course the individual cannot conceivably influence or when the individual has no special access to predictive data. Another worry relates to depressive predictive certainty, which, it will be recalled, describes how pessimistic predictions are held with increasing conviction as negative mood deepens.[35] It is known, too, that depressed assessments can pertain to a wide range of contingencies.[36] It seems doubtful that depressives accurately perceive a general deterioration in states of affairs, warranting an ever-more negative affective response. Rather, a more parsimonious and more likely explanation is that the negativity of predictions is, at least partially, a function of depressed affect.

Depressive realism has also been questioned by empirical findings suggesting the phenomenon applies only when nondepressed control groups demonstrate overconfidence in relation to a study task. Fu and colleagues hypothesized that when tasks resulted in realistic or underconfident assessments by controls, the pessimistic evaluations of depressed subjects would be unrealistic.[37] They asked depressed and nondepressed subjects to judge the comparative size of two objects, match flags with their respective countries, and indicate which of two inventions took place earlier. Subjects were then required to rate their performance. The authors found that *both* groups underestimated their performance, with the depressed group doing so to a slightly greater extent. There was no evidence of more realistic estimations in the depressed group. These findings echo those of Dunning and Story, who assessed depressed and nondepressed college students on the accuracy of predictions made during an academic semester.[38] Actions and events that were assessed included dropping a course, beginning a major relationship, and being the victim of a crime. The investigators found that depressed students were, overall, less realistic in their predictions. More recently, Carson and colleagues found little evidence for realistic assessments by depressed participants on a contingency judgment task.[39] The authors suggested that a limitation in earlier studies with contrary findings was a failure to utilize participants with "bona fide" major depression. Thus, many previous studies used students who, while demonstrating dysphoria on self-report measures, had not been clinically diagnosed with the more serious major depressive disorder. As a result, the enhanced predictive accuracy of dysphoric participants may have limited applicability to those with major depression, who were the exclusive subject of the present study.

These data, and the evidence for negative biases, suggest that predictions in depression are, in the main, excessively pessimistic. The case for depressive realism is unpersuasive. Having established the empirical basis for negative information-processing biases, it is now possible to consider their effect on the autonomy of those with depression.

4.3 Information-Processing Biases and the Erosion of Autonomy in Depression

In chapter 3, I argued that the agent who holds justified beliefs about the evidential value of his or her affective response is more autonomous in dealing with the affective trigger. Now I will argue that negative affect in depression has poor evidential value. That is, negative affect tends to promote the holding of unjustified beliefs in relation to its triggering event. This property alone, I argue, is sufficient to antagonize autonomy. However, I will also show that many depressed people do not comprehend the poor evidential value of affect in this disorder and, therefore, often take dubious cognitions at face value. This failure of reflective awareness heightens their liability to form unjustified beliefs about the affective trigger. These combined effects, I conclude, seriously threaten autonomy in those with depression.

4.3.1 Negative Affect Undermines Autonomy in Depression

An understanding of negative biases provides good reason to be cautious about the evidential value of affect in depression. Consider the following example. Penelope, in the midst of a depressive episode, is at work when her colleague Harriet, who is looking steadfastly at the floor, passes her in a corridor. Penelope forms the view that Harriet has ignored her. She further concludes that Harriet is avoiding her and dislikes her. However, it seems clear that Harriet could have a myriad of reasons to appear self-focused and remote. She might have work or family problems that have nothing to do with Penelope. What is salient is that a depressed Penelope is *more likely* to make a negative assessment than if she were not depressed and that her conclusions are less likely to be veridical.

I will now advance two claims to show how Penelope's depressed affect undermines the autonomy of her subsequent decisions. The first claim is that some fact in relation to the belief, "Harriet is ignoring me and dislikes me" is material to Penelope. The second claim is that depressed affect makes it improbable that Penelope will hold justified beliefs about that material fact. Support for the first claim comes from a central tenet of appraisal theory; affect tends to arise when the agent has a principal goal or interest at stake in the eliciting event. That the corridor encounter was sufficient to evoke affect suggests that Penelope has a strong investment in her relationship with Harriet. If a *stranger* staring at the floor passed her in the corridor, an affective response would be less likely. The interest at stake in the relationship might relate to a common project the pair is working on, or Harriet might be more senior and a promotion might hinge on her endorsement. Perhaps Harriet is held in high esteem and great value is placed on her approval. A perceived threat to any of these interests could elicit an affective response. The *fact* of an *actual* threat to each of these interests is plausibly material to Penelope.

Support for the second claim—that Penelope is unlikely to hold justified beliefs in relation to the material fact—comes from the empirical data on biases in depression. Negative biases increase the likelihood that inaccurate, pessimistic predictions will be made. Further, depressive predictive certainty shows negative biases to become more pronounced as depressive symptoms worsen. These data suggest that Penelope's interpretation of events will be unrealistically negative. Thoughts like "Harriet dislikes me," "I am a failure," "I will never be promoted," and "Our project will collapse" are typical of those experienced in depression yet are probably mistaken. Facts about the encounter with Harriet are material to Harriet, but negative affect makes it unlikely that she will hold justified beliefs in relation to those facts. Depressed affect has a strong potential to erode the autonomy of Penelope's subsequent decisions.

4.3.2 Failure to Hold Justified Beliefs about Negative Affect Undermines Autonomy in Depression

However, a failure to hold justified beliefs *about* negative affect also undermines autonomy in depression. Two claims support this contention. First, the propensity of depressed affect to mislead is likely to be material to the depressed person. Second, the person with depression is unlikely to hold justified beliefs about the deceptive nature of negative affect.

The first claim derives, again, from appraisal theory. Events that trigger affect usually impact on the agent's dominant interests, so facts about them are likely to be material. It follows that information about an *obstacle* to gleaning those facts would also be material, especially if that knowledge helped the agent circumvent the hurdle. Depressed affect engenders false beliefs about triggering events and so impedes the understanding of material facts. Moreover, it is an impediment that, I will show, can be overcome. The deceptive nature of negative affect is, therefore, likely to be material to the person with depression. Thus, facts about the distressing encounter with Harriet are material to Penelope, and negative affect has led her to draw improbable conclusions about their relationship. As a result, it is also likely to be material to Penelope that *negative affect is misleading*, and her response to Harriet will be more autonomous with that understanding. Thus, if Penelope is alert to negative affect as a confounding influence on her appraisal of Harriet's behavior, she is positioned to engage in a more systematic analysis of the incident. She might, for example, muster the resolve to give equal consideration to, and evaluate, alternative explanations for Harriet's actions. She could also make tactful approaches to other staff or even approach Harriet herself to determine whether her suspicions are misplaced or well-founded. This empirical approach is more reliable in the presence of biased affective evaluations and carries a greater likelihood of arriving at justified beliefs about the encounter.

As explained in chapter 2, sound epistemic appraisals further autonomy by prompting actions that are more likely to cohere with the agent's values, raising the chances that relevant interests will be protected and facilitating effective control in challenging circumstances. Imagine that Penelope's inquiry reveals Harriet has recently separated from her spouse and is having difficulty coping. It would be reasonable to expect this to be a primary influence on her current behavior. Taking this into account, Penelope's ensuing decisions will conceivably orient more toward maintaining the course of their collaborative efforts while adopting a stance of deference and understanding with respect to her colleague's misfortune. This result accords with the broader value she places on academic achievement, is most favorable to the specific interests inherent in the joint endeavor, and allows greater control over a potentially adverse incident. Justified beliefs about the poor evidential value of affect in depression have promoted justified beliefs about the affective trigger, as well as a more autonomous response to it. An alternative scenario is that Penelope heeds those cognitions that are reinforced by negative affect. Working on the assumptions that Harriet's behavior signals a dislike for her, corroborates suspicions of her own ineptitude, and is a harbinger of ill for their work, Penelope might respond very differently. She could avoid work by ringing in sick. She might make excuses to Harriet and gradually withdraw from their academic partnership. She could refrain from applying for a promotion, ensuring that she will be overlooked during the next round, and so on. These actions derive from unjustified beliefs about material matters and frustrate Penelope's autonomous response to the encounter with Harriet. The diminished autonomy evidenced in her behavior is antithetical to the values, interests, and control just delineated.

Now I want to substantiate the second claim, which is that people with depression are unlikely to hold justified beliefs about the deceptive properties of negative affect. This claim is supported by a prima facie contention; if depressed individuals held justified beliefs about negative affect and its biases, it is unlikely they would generate the pessimistic predictions that typify depression. Worsening depression leads to a correspondingly greater conviction with which negative sentiments are held. It is difficult to see how pessimism could be embraced with such certainty yet coexist with skepticism about the veracity of depressive cognitions. Given the ubiquity of pessimism in depression, it seems clear that few depressed people hold realistic beliefs about the confounding nature of negative affect. This claim is further supported by a principal approach used in the treatment of depression in cognitive therapy. "Mindfulness" teaches the depressed person to "stand back" from, and adopt a "decentered" or "distanced" approach to negative thoughts and feelings.[40] As Teasdale and colleagues describe it, individuals learn to relate to these mental events as "passing thoughts and feelings that may or may not have some truth in them" rather than as "the reality by which I am condemned."[41] This altered mode of perceiving thoughts and feelings in depression is termed "meta-cognitive awareness." The therapeutic mechanism of mindfulness makes an assumption that depressed patients see their negative thoughts and feelings as "reality" and not as a manifestation of biased thought processes. The therapeutic effectiveness of mindfulness[42] suggests the assumption is a correct one. Although indirect evidence, this observation supports the idea that depressed individuals, mostly, fail to hold justified beliefs about the unreliable nature of negative affect. The poor evidence of negative affect in depression is material, and failure to comprehend it works against autonomy.

4.4   Stress and Depression

I now want to develop the second strand of the argument that depression undermines autonomy. My contention is that a failure to hold justified beliefs about the action of stressors poses a considerable threat to the autonomy of those with depression. In order to build this case, it is first necessary to outline the empirical findings that link stressors and depression.

4.4.1   Psychosocial Stressors Trigger Depression

The influential "diathesis–stress" model holds that depression manifests in predisposed individuals presented with a sufficiently stressful stimulus.[43] Empirical evidence suggests that psychosocial stressors are identifiable triggers in a significant percentage of depressive episodes. For example, Kendler and colleagues studied depression in around 2,000 members of the Virginia Twin Registry.[44] They found that stressful life events were "strongly and significantly associated with the risk of onset of depressive episodes."[45] The researchers concluded that 65 percent of associations between stressful life events and depression were causal associations. Stressful life events included, among others, job loss, marital separation, and financial difficulties. Kessler arrived at a similar conclusion in a review article on data linking stress and depression:

The evidence reviewed . . . clearly shows that inventories of stressful events predict subsequent depression. A smaller number of controlled comparative studies of people exposed to single major life events provide strong evidence that at least part of this association is due to events causing depression.[46]

In a comprehensive review, Hammen noted research suggesting up to 80 percent of depressive episodes are preceded by major life events and concluded there is a "robust and causal association between stressful life events and major depressive episodes."[47]

A connection between stressful life events and depression is further supported by the observation that contingencies promoting depression tend to be nonrandom. That is, the kinds of circumstances that are associated with new-onset and recurrent depression are largely predictable and conform to two categories. The first comprises a threat to the individual's sense of power, manifesting as feelings of defeat or humiliation. The other involves threats to affiliation, that is, to the individual's close personal relationships. These are expressed as perceptions of social rejection and being shunned or as a feeling of loss.[48] Empirical data support the intuition that the association is not merely a correlation but that a causal link exists between these kinds of occurrences and subsequent depressive episodes.[49]

However, it is important to consider evidence questioning the significance of stress in the etiology of depression. Some research suggests that stress might be particularly important in causing a first episode of depression, with later episodes being less dependent on the presence of environmental triggers.[50] The conceptual basis for this so-called "kindling" model of depression derives from electrophysiological experiments in animals.[51] In these studies, small electrical stimuli that did not initially cause seizures were found to do so after repeated delivery. Eventually, seizures became "autonomous," occurring in the absence of any stimulus. The depression analog or "stress sensitization" account sees the depressogenic potency of stressful life events increasing as the agent's exposure to them mounts. Supporting the kindling hypothesis, Kendler and colleagues found that as the number of depressive episodes increases, the likelihood that a causative stressor will be identified decreases.[52] Specifically, the investigators found that, over the first nine episodes, stressors of ever-diminishing potency could trigger depression, but beyond the ninth episode the relationship did not alter. It remains unclear whether tenth and later episodes no longer require stress as an etiological agent or whether the individual becomes so sensitized that depression is brought on by very minor adversity.[53] If the kindling account is correct, it is important to acknowledge its possible implications for the argument that follows. I argue that an understanding of the stress–depression link is material to the autonomous decision making of depressed people. If, for some experiencing multiple recurrences, stressors are not discernible beyond the ninth episode, the importance of this link may be lessened. As a result, the argument put forward has particular relevance for those experiencing initial episodes of depression.

A second challenge to the contention that stressors are depressogenic is the observation that some depression seems to have a more "endogenous" or "biological" character. This subcategory is termed "melancholic depression" and has traditionally been thought to occur independent of the action of stressors. Melancholic depression is characterized by a loss of pleasure in all, or almost all, activities and by psychomotor changes, which can include a slowing of movements and mental processes or, conversely, agitation.[54] The few studies addressing the claim that melancholia is unrelated to stressors have found some, but not conclusive, support for it. For example, while Mitchell and colleagues found stressful events were more likely to precede first episodes of depression in those with a nonmelancholic subtype,[55] an earlier study by Brown and colleagues found no significant difference in the frequency of stressful events between patients with endogenous and nonendogenous depression.[56] Moreover, a recent study by Harkness and Monroe found that women with melancholic depression were *more* sensitive to the effects of psychosocial stressors than those suffering the nonmelancholic variety.[57] In addition, controversy exists as to the responsiveness of melancholic depression to psychotherapy. There is a long-standing view that melancholia is more resistant to psychotherapy and more receptive to medication.[58] However, that standpoint is challenged in a recent study by Luty and colleagues, who found that melancholic and nonmelancholic depression were equally responsive to CBT and IPT.[59]

Aside from the equivocation concerning a role for stress, and the effectiveness of psychotherapy, it should be noted that melancholic depression is a relatively uncommon subtype. Its lifetime prevalence is around 1 percent to 2 percent for both men and women, compared to a lifetime prevalence for nonmelancholic depression of around 17 percent for men and 25 percent for women.[60] As melancholia comprises only a small minority of cases, it will not significantly alter the depression demographic encountered by doctors. However, it has relevance for the argument being developed here, in that doctors need to be aware of this category and be alert to its potential to be less responsive to psychotherapy than more common subtypes.

4.4.2 A Neurobiological Mechanism for Stressors Triggering Depression

Researchers have sought a neurobiological explanation for a connection between stress and depression. Increasing evidence points to a mediating role for the hormone cortisol. It is known that sustained stress increases the release of cortisol from the adrenal gland and that high cortisol levels can damage the hippocampus, a structure in the brain's emotional center, the limbic system.[61] Adults with major depression have a greater incidence of hippocampal atrophy,[62,63] and around half of people diagnosed with depression have excessive activation of cortisol production.[64] Robert Sapolsky, an authority on this subject, has concluded that, on available data, stress and elevated cortisol levels inhibit the growth of nerves in the hippocampus.[65] The hippocampus also acts to inhibit cortisol secretion,[66] so damage to it reduces inhibition, further elevating cortisol. This might contribute to a positive feedback loop, which sustains detrimental effects on the hippocampus. Stressful life events are associated with increased cortisol secretion in both healthy subjects[67] and those with depression.[68] These data suggest that cortisol elevations from stressful life events may cause depression, a conclusion that at least one reviewer affirms.[69] However, no study to date has conclusively substantiated this claim.

A further mechanism by which cortisol elevations might trigger depression relates to serotonin metabolism. Serotonin is a chemical messenger in the brain that has been implicated in emotion regulation. Prolonged rises in cortisol levels can reduce both serotonin and the sensitivity of receptors to its action.[70] The role of serotonin in the etiology of depression is complex. A respected hypothesis is that lowered serotonin leads to reduced levels of another protein, brain derived neurotrophic factor (BDNF).[71] In animal models, BDNF levels in the hippocampus are diminished by stress and cortisol,[72] and reduced hippocampal BDNF has been found in postmortem studies of depressed patients.[73] BDNF deficiency is thought to cause hippocampal atrophy,[74] so stress and cortisol might trigger depression by this route also.

Evidence points to cortisol as a mediator of the depressogenic effects of stress, with damage to the hippocampus presenting as a likely neuroanatomical correlate of that process. While these empirical data remain suggestive rather than definitive, their importance for the argument to come is that they lend further credibility to the existence of a stress–depression link. As a result, they heighten the salience of an understanding of causal stressors as elemental to the autonomy of those with depression.

4.4.3 The Role of Diathesis in Depression

It must be remembered that, in depression, the stressor lies on one side of the diathesis–stress dichotomy. The diathesis–stress model proposes that, for depression to manifest, stressors need to act in the setting of an appropriately vulnerable individual. A range of contingencies renders individuals susceptible to developing depression. The most significant correlations have emerged between early life adversity and later depression. Kendler and colleagues have shown that, in women, childhood sexual abuse, childhood parental loss, a disturbed family environment,[75] and genetic predisposition all contribute to an increased risk of later life depression.[76] The same investigators have collected data supporting similar conclusions in men.[77] It is hypothesized that risk factors in early life predict the emergence of a depressogenic "cognitive style" in adolescence and adulthood.[78] Most research has focused on negative attributional style as a response mode that heightens the risk of stressor exposure's being translated into a depressive episode.[79] Negative attributional style, discussed in more detail in the final section of this chapter, involves excessive self-blame for poor outcomes and unwarranted predictions of subsequent unpleasant occurrences.

Given the evidence for heritability in depression, research has also aimed to identify a genetic abnormality in those predisposed to the disorder. Several studies suggest that genes coding for a protein that modifies the brain's utilization of serotonin might be involved. The serotonin transporter, or 5-HTT gene,[80] is responsible for the manufacture of a protein that enhances uptake of serotonin. The gene has long and short alleles. Individuals with two short alleles make much less of the transporter protein than those with two long alleles, or those with one long and one short.[81] Caspi and colleagues found that individuals with two short alleles were more likely to display suicidality, and to be diagnosed with depression after stressful events, than those who were homozygous for the long allele.[82] Kendler and colleagues broadly replicated these findings.[83] However, authors of a meta-analysis of 11 related studies were less sanguine. They found there was "no conclusive evidence suggesting that variations at genes coding for 5-HT receptors or 5HTT may confer susceptibility for [major depressive disorder]."[84] More recently, a meta-analysis of 14 studies affirmed that stressful life events have a "potent relationship with risk of depression" but found no evidence that 5HTT genotype altered risk for major depression beyond that associated with stressful life events.[85]

I bring out the importance of diathesis for the current argument in chapter 6. There, I outline an objection that cognitive vulnerability diminishes the material significance of an understanding of depressive triggers, a claim that I reject. Now, though, I want to argue that failure to appreciate the role of stressors undermines the autonomy of those with depression.

4.5   Failure to Hold Justified Beliefs about the Role of Stressors Undermines Autonomy in Depression

The evidence adduced suggests that stressors can precipitate depressive episodes. In this section, I aim to substantiate two claims. The first claim is that facts concerning the triggering role of stressors are likely to be material to the depressed person. The second claim is that people with depression often fail to hold justified beliefs about triggering stressors. These claims will ground a conclusion that failure to hold justified beliefs about psychosocial stressors undermines the autonomy of important, related decisions in depression.

4.5.1   The Materiality of Psychosocial Stressors

In chapter 3, I argued that affect indicates triggering events to be pertinent to the agent's interests, and so facts about those events are likely to be material to the agent. I have shown that, in many instances of depression, stressors have been sufficient to cause that affective response. It follows that stressors probably relate to the depressed person's important interests and that facts surrounding them are material. When the nature of triggering events is considered, it is not difficult to see why this might be so. In the study by Kendler and colleagues, described earlier, psychosocial stressors causing depression included assault, rape, mugging, divorce, broken engagement, and breakup of a romantic relationship.[86] Also implicated were financial problems, housing problems, serious illness or injury, job loss, serious problems at work, legal problems, serious marital problems, and being robbed.[87]

It is clear that all of these classes of stressor impact on important interests and, in virtue of that property, understanding their significant facets would be material to the agent's corresponding decisions. For example, the ramifications of financial difficulties for people with a mortgage, or who are raising a family, make details of causes, effects, and solutions necessary to protect the interests at stake. Because even small variations in these details carry serious potential repercussions for the agent's interests, the details are materially significant. However, there is a further category of information concerning stressors that is likely to be material to the depressed person. I refer to the capacity of stressors to *precipitate depression*. I premise this claim on the observation that a depressed response to a stressor will, in all likelihood, set back the person's interests in relation to it. Goal-directed behavior entails focused, motivated decisions and action. Depression, characterized by poor concentration, diminished energy, and impaired decision making, typically works against the fulfillment of goals and interests. Drawing a connection between depression and stressors emphasizes the urgency with which a new approach to those events is required. Thus, when financial problems trigger depression, it is material not just that the individual's mode of response has hastened his or her economic woes but that it has led to a depression that greatly hinders the individual's setting things right.

Of course, depressed people do not only have interest in addressing triggering events; they also wish to be rid of depression. However, an understanding of the role of stressors is important here as well. There are good reasons for people to be apprised of causative factors in illness, not least of which is that understanding etiological agents can assist recovery. The asthmatic who smokes can use knowledge of the link between cigarettes and respiratory illness to hasten recuperation. Even if he or she ultimately chooses to continue smoking, understanding its effects remains material to the individual's future decisions about managing asthma. Similarly, the depressed person who comprehends the role of stressors is apprised of facts that are material not just in dealing with those stressors but also to the ongoing management of his or her depression.

It is plausible, too, that the fact of a stressor–depression relationship might retain materiality for the depressed person even if a causal relationship were not determined with certainty in that person's specific case. To see this, it is helpful to understand the stressor as a *risk factor* for depression in those with the appropriate vulnerability. Informing patients of risk factors for a current illness is, quite rightly, accepted health care practice. Consider the analogy of a company director who sees the family physician for follow-up after a heart attack. Emerging evidence suggests that stress increases heart attack risk through a raft of effects, including greater propensity for blood to clot.[88,89] Thus, stress is likely to be a risk factor for heart disease in a similar category to smoking, diabetes, and high blood pressure. Even though a causal relationship between a stressful job and coronary disease might not be established with certainty in this instance, being apprised of the risk permits informed choices about whether, or how best, to continue in that role. For the depressed person, understanding the stressor–depression relationship is material for parallel reasons. That knowledge furthers informed decisions about risking potentially depressogenic exposures to stress at work and in a range of other contexts. In what follows, I argue that depressed people frequently do not grasp the significance of stressors and that autonomy suffers as a result. It will then be possible to make conclusions about the evidence afforded by affect in relation to stressors in depression, and its relevance to autonomy.

4.5.2   Failure to Hold Justified Beliefs about Stressors in Depression
In this section I present an argument in two parts. In the first part, I argue that many depressed people fail to understand that a connection between psychosocial stressors and depression exists. In the second part, I show that, even when the depressed person appreciates that connection, his or her interpretation of it is often flawed. Both contingencies, I will conclude, make it improbable that depressed people will hold justified beliefs about the material role of stressors in their illness.

Justified Psychosocial Beliefs Displaced by Unjustified Biological Beliefs about Depression Causation   There is evidence that at least a third of people believe depression results from altered brain chemistry that is primary and independent of the effect of life events. In a study of 2,000 German nationals, randomly sampled from private households, Matschinger and Angermeyer found that 25 percent of respondents favored "brain disorder" and 37 percent cited "heredity" as likely causes of depression.[90] In the same survey, around 60 percent thought that "weak mental constitution" or "unstable personality" was to blame. However, 75 to 80 percent did cite situational stressors such as isolation, unemployment, and occupational or family stress as causes. The same researchers conducted a larger study seven years later, surveying 5,000 people.[91] They found a similar prevalence of beliefs about situational stressors but an increase in beliefs about biomedical origins of depression, with 41 percent of respondents citing "brain disease" as causal. In Switzerland, Lauber and colleagues also investigated general views on depression, interviewing 876 people. Fifty-six percent believed family difficulties were responsible, and 32 percent cited occupational stress as a likely cause. Around one-third of respondents regarded depression as "biological" or "disease-related" in origin.[92] In the United States, Blumner and Marcus analyzed data from the General Social Survey, which contains interview responses from adults in private households. They found the number of respondents believing that depression results from a "chemical imbalance in the brain" increased in that country from 71 percent in 1996 to 84 percent in 2006.[93] In the same study, 94 percent of respondents endorsed "stressful circumstances" as contributing to depression, with minimal change in that figure over the studied decade.

A number of studies have examined beliefs about etiology in those who have experienced depression. Srinivasan and colleagues asked 102 people with depression to evaluate statements that included the following:

• I have a biological abnormality (for example, chemical or hormonal imbalance).
• The way I evaluate or think about my experiences caused my depression. [This question assesses "cognitive style"]
• Stress and negative life experiences caused my depression.[94]

Responses were rated on a Likert scale, with 0 indicating "not at all" and 10 indicating "definitely." The authors found the mean score for biological abnormality to be 4.48; for cognitive style, 5.61; and for stress or negative life events, 6.55. In a smaller study, Brown and colleagues examined the "personal illness models" of 41 primary care patients with depression.[95] Again, the findings follow a consistent trend with 68 percent of respondents citing stress as causative in their illness and 32 percent attributing their depression to "medical illness." Depression here was thought of as a medical illness itself, not as a reaction to a coexisting medical condition, which featured as a separate questionnaire item.

If these studies are representative, at least one-third of people diagnosed with depression are likely to believe their illness to be "biological," a figure that, accepting the data of Blumner and Marcus, may be significantly higher in the United States. I want to suggest that it is plausible, too, that many in this group will see their depression as bearing little relation to the action of environmental stressors. While it is acknowledged that at least two-thirds of depressed people are likely to nominate psychosocial stressors as contributory, there is reason to think that, for many, biological and psychosocial beliefs about etiology will not overlap. Warrant for this view stems from the push, prevalent in the United States, to frame etiology as biological in order to reduce the social stigma attached to mental illness.

For example, the Indiana branch of Mental Health America, a national advocacy organization, asserts, "Depression is more than 'the blues,' it cannot be willed or wished away. It is not a sign of personal weakness. It is a flaw in chemistry not character."[96] As Deacon and Baird explain, the rationale for this approach is that labeling depression as biological or "brain based" divorces the disorder from the individual's personality or volition and places it outside his or her direct control.[97] If individuals cannot be "blamed" for their illness, they are less liable, some argue, to experience stereotyping and discriminatory treatment. As the authors note, this view has found wide favor, despite empirical evidence now questioning its legitimacy.[98] In their own study, Deacon and Baird found that undergraduate students who favored a chemical imbalance explanation for depression were less likely to perceive psychosocial interventions to be effective.[99] This finding describes a tension between biological and psychosocial explanations for depression, which suggests they are seen to compete with, rather than complement, one another. I want to argue now that most depressed people who see their illness as biologically based, with a minimal role for triggering stressors, are mistaken.

Recall that melancholic depression, the category thought most likely to stem from biological causes alone, accounts for only 1 to 2 percent of cases. On this estimate, a significant proportion of the one-third of depressed people with biological beliefs about etiology will, in fact, have discernible triggering stressors. This claim derives from Kendler's figure that around 65 percent of depressive episodes are stressor related and the plausible assumption that depressed people with biological beliefs remain well-described by this epidemiology. If biological beliefs exist without an understanding of the psychosocial dimension of depression, many in this group will, therefore, fail to hold justified beliefs about the role of stressors in their illness. Moreover, those with melancholia itself might also be found to have precipitating stressors if the findings of Harkness and Monroe, cited earlier, are robust.[100] These investigators concluded that melancholic depression might be *more sensitive* to stressors, with minor adversity having greater depressogenic potential in this category than in nonmelancholic depression. In this case, some with melancholia who hold biological beliefs, and who eschew or fail to be aware of psychosocial causes of depression, may hold unjustified beliefs about the etiological role of stressors in their own depression.

I describe a significant proportion of depressed people with biological beliefs, who do not appreciate the role of stressors, and who therefore fail to hold justified beliefs about the cause of their depression. It is reasonable to conclude that, if biological and environmental explanations for depression compete, reinforcement of a biological model will occur at the expense of justified beliefs about stressor causation. I now want to illustrate a prevailing medical environment that favors pharmacotherapy in depression and which, in so doing, works to strengthen biological beliefs and to reduce an appreciation for psychosocial causes. This approach, I will show, works to further undermine the autonomy of people with depression.

In Australia, around 80 percent of people diagnosed with depression by a primary care practitioner receive antidepressant medication.[101] In 2004–2005, primary care physicians wrote 11,248,200 prescriptions for antidepressants, up from 7,465,919 in 1999–2000.[102] The total cost to the Australian Pharmaceutical Benefits Scheme in 2004–2005 for antidepressant prescriptions in general practice was AU $482,090,000, up from AU $276,135,000 in 1999–2000.[103] The number of people who see a primary care doctor for depression and are treated with proven forms of psychotherapy—cognitive behavior, interpersonal, or problem-solving therapies—cannot be precisely ascertained from the most comprehensive report available.[104] However, it is no greater than 25 percent, and probably significantly less. This figure derives from the observation that around 50 percent of people with depression seen in primary care are given a "clinical treatment," and roughly half of clinical treatments involve psychological counseling.[105] However, it is unclear from the report precisely what percentage of counseling comprises psychotherapy of proven efficacy in depression.

Figures from the United States also show high rates of antidepressant use for major depressive disorder. In that country, the percentage of adults using antidepressants more than tripled between 1994 and 2002 from 2.5 to 8 percent.[106] This comprised a rise from 3.3 to 10.6 percent among women and from 1.6 to 5.2 percent among men. Between 2002 and 2005 antidepressant prescriptions increased by over 10 percent from 154.1 million to 169.9 million[107] with spending on the top two antidepressants alone, Paxil and Zoloft, totaling U.S. $4.4 billion in 2002.[108] Estimates of depressed outpatients who receive antidepressants range from 52 to 79 percent, with 27 to 60 percent undergoing some form of psychotherapy.[109,110] It is unclear from the relevant studies what proportion of psychotherapy instances included a validated treatment such as CBT, IPT, or problem-solving therapy, but it is likely to be only a fraction of the cited overall therapy percentages. For example, in the study by Olfson and colleagues, "psychotherapy" covered any treatment the respondent health care provider would classify as "psychotherapy or mental health counseling." Given that over 400 categories of psychotherapy have been identified, there is great potential for the delivery of therapy that lacks clinical trial validation.

These figures describe a significant increase in the prescribing of antidepressants in primary care in recent years. They also demonstrate an approach to the treatment of depression that could reasonably be seen as reinforcing erroneous beliefs about its etiology. For example, a minority of cases of depression can be attributed to primary changes in brain chemistry, yet a substantial majority of depressed individuals in primary care receive antidepressants. Conversely, at least two-thirds of depressive episodes can be linked to triggering stressors, yet the therapies that specifically address such stressors, and are of proven efficacy, count for less than 25 percent of treatments in Australia with, as discussed, similar figures probably applying in the United States. Of course, ADM might deliver effective symptom relief in stressor-associated depression, and psychotherapy may have some benefits in biological depression. However, at issue here are the implications of a dominant cultural treatment ethos on patient beliefs about causes of depression. Indeed, emerging data support the intuition that promulgation of ADM for depression management fosters acceptance of a biological explanation for depression. France and colleagues surveyed 262 psychology undergraduates in the midwestern United States.[111] They found that 92 percent of respondents had heard the explanation of depression as an "imbalance of chemicals in the brain" and, of those, 89 percent had encountered this information through television, most likely in the form of direct-to-consumer advertising (DTCA) of ADM. Of this cohort, 54 percent agreed with the statement "Depression is primarily caused by an imbalance of chemicals in the brain." While the study design did not permit conclusions to be drawn about DTCA as an explicit cause of participants' beliefs, it seems reasonable to infer that it was at least contributory. Also in the United States, Leykin and colleagues evaluated the beliefs of depressed patients before and after treatment with either cognitive therapy or pharmacotherapy.[112] They found those successfully treated with cognitive therapy to have reduced beliefs about biological causation of depression. Conversely, patients who successfully received pharmacotherapy had a reduction in so-called "characterological" beliefs—that cognitions, thoughts, and "seeing things in a depressive way" are significant contributors to depressive symptomatology. The authors suggest that belief in the efficacy of a particular treatment reinforces related beliefs about etiology. They further conjecture this dichotomous view to stem from patients' seeing characterological and biological reasons for depression as competing.

Biological causation might not simply be tacitly promoted through the focus on pharmacotherapy for depression. There is evidence that such beliefs are also widespread in members of the medical profession who inculcate patients with this conception. In a small qualitative study of physicians' beliefs about the nature of depression, statements that reflect a biological approach were frequent.[113] Of 20 physicians surveyed, one expressed the view that depression was "no different to diabetes," an analogy that was endorsed by a further eight physicians. In the same study, a physician described depression as a "neurotransmitter deficiency," and another told patients that antidepressants would correct a "chemical problem in [their] nervous systems."[114] In Western Canada, Schreiber and Hartrick conducted a qualitative study of 43 women with depression and found that all interviewees, in varying degrees, invoked biochemical or genetic explanations for their depression.[115] Moreover, it was generally proffered that the treating physician had been the source of information concerning this explanatory model. Of further interest, some embraced a biomedical model after treatment with ADM and subsequently revoked a long-standing acceptance of psychosocial causes of the disorder. As the authors explain,

[i]n essence, the women used the BEM [biomedical explanatory model] in a way that reduced the multidimensionality of the depression experience to a single (bio-chemical) phenomenon. . . . Psychosocial factors that were sufficiently important for the women to emphasise when describing their depression faded away as the BEM gained ascendance. . . . The BEM obscured the possibility of understanding depression as a relational phenomenon.[116]

These data gain significance when it is remembered that around 75 percent of people with depression who seek treatment attend their general practitioner[117] with four-fifths of these receiving ADM.[118] It is improbable that doctors who treat a high percentage of their depressed patients with ADM, and withhold psychotherapy, would educate these people about the causal role of stressors in depression. It is equally improbable that depressed patients would willingly accept antidepressants without therapy while simultaneously understanding that stress causes depression and that psychotherapy can address both issues. A rational conclusion, therefore, is that a prevailing preference for a drug-based approach to treatment contributes to depressed patients' holding biological beliefs about depression causation. As outlined earlier in this chapter, it is now beyond dispute that changes in the brain's neurotransmitters, nerve growth factors, and even anatomy are instrumental to the development of depressive symptoms. However, it is critical information that such changes can be brought about by identifiable, contextual, environmental factors and that stressors conform to this class of stimulus. It is equally critical that non-pharmacological treatments such as CBT are not only effective in depression but, as I outline in chapter 6 (section 6.5.2), are also likely to address its accompanying neurobiological derangements.

Other studies do affirm recognition by general practitioners that stressors play an important role in depression.[119] However, many doctors feel pressured to prescribe antidepressants because psychology services are inadequate to cope with demand. Commenting on delayed patient access to psychologists, one GP said the following:

It's about four months at the moment. So that's a problem. A lot of people end up being put on medication. Perhaps if they could see a psychologist in two weeks then they wouldn't need medication.[120]

General practitioners also face considerable time pressures in their daily schedule, so consultations for people with depression are often short, and the less time-consuming option of pharmacotherapy becomes attractive to the physician. In the United Kingdom, mean primary care consultation time is around 8 minutes, with some practitioners extending that to 20 minutes for first consultations with depressed patients.[121] However, in one study, follow-up appointments of the standard length, 5–10 minutes, were deemed sufficient to adequately manage depression.[122] But these consultation periods are too short to address the kinds of stressors that are implicated in depressive illness. Even a standard course of problem-solving therapy requires an initial one-hour session followed by five half hour sessions,[123] and a single course of CBT involves a total of 16 hours' contact time with the therapist.

There is a medical environment of high antidepressant prescribing rates, short consultation times, and relatively low rates of referral for validated psychotherapy. A prevalent ethos among physicians that depression has a biological basis makes it less likely they will encourage depressed people to seek to identify and address stressors. Many patients might also form the view, after medical consultation, that stressors do not play a significant role in depression. Accepting this interpretation, it is probable that many depressed people will not hold justified beliefs about the causal role of psychosocial stressors in their illness. I concede the data presented here suggesting the majority of people with depression are likely to cite stressors as probable causes. However, unless a treating physician corroborates that belief, and the nature of the stressor is elucidated, then it is plausible that such a belief will merely remain a suspicion rather than being held with conviction. It is the *fact* of a connection between stressors and depression that is material to the depressed person. Unless the individual is prepared to conduct his or her own research, confirmation of that material fact necessarily comes from an informed physician. Without physician input, it is difficult to ensure that a patient has the degree of factual understanding necessary to satisfy an autonomy requirement.

Negative Attributional Style Fosters Unjustified Beliefs about Psychosocial Stressors Yet, there is a final important reason to hold that the depressed person might fail to accurately appreciate the role of psychosocial stressors. Negative information-processing biases have a strong impact on the way those with depression interpret stressors. As mentioned earlier in this chapter, negative attributional style is a biased thinking pattern common in depression. This "dysfunctional inferential style" leads individuals to "characteristically explain negative events in terms of internal, global and stable causes."[124] "Internal" refers to the observation that depressed people commonly see themselves as the primary cause of negative life events. "Global" describes how they see those events as triggering many other negative outcomes. "Stable" denotes the perception that resulting dire effects will endure.[125] For example, a depressed person evincing this cognitive style might, on receiving an unfriendly greeting from an acquaintance, believe his or her own behavior has caused offense, surmise that other people will also respond hostilely, and predict this state of affairs will persist for the foreseeable future. Negative attributional style is a cognitive vulnerability comprising a major element of the depression diathesis. Moreover, there is solid evidence that it increases depression risk by heightening "reactivity" to stressors.[126] Thus, when negative self-attributions are prominent in a stressor response, depression is more likely to result.[127]

Because negative attributional style is a product of biased information processing, it tends to give rise to unrealistically negative interpretations of events.[128] Negative attributional style suggests that even when depressed people identify stressors, there is a good chance they will make inaccurate appraisals. Thus, a stressor might not be seen as inherently taxing, and its ill effects might instead be blamed on the individual's own perceived deficiencies. Stressors might also be seen as irremediable and overwhelming when, in fact, problem-focused approaches can be effective in addressing them.[129] These observations indicate strong potential for depressed people to lack justified beliefs about the role of stressors in their illness.

Moreover, there is cause to believe that depressed affect may be a mediator of negative attributional style. This claim occurs amid debate on whether negative attributional style is an ever-present trait placing vulnerable individuals at risk of depression during stressor exposure or whether negative attributions are "state-like" and mood-dependent, only becoming operative during periods of negative affect. The latter view, termed the "mood state hypothesis," suggests that while a negative cognitive style is integral to personality, it remains latent until the catalyst of negative mood causes it to manifest.[130] Supporting this hypothesis, the cognitive vulnerability of depressed people reduces when they return to "euthymia," or normal mood.[131] Thus, when depression is remitted or recovered, individuals do not demonstrate the described negative attributions. Recent corroboration also comes from Ball and colleagues, who found that attributional style correlates more closely to extant negative mood than to either a history of or current diagnosis of depression.[132] Some research also suggests cognitive vulnerability might comprise both "trait" and "state" components.[133] Overall, it is reasonable to conclude from these data that negative affect plays a significant role as mediator of negative attributions.

4.5.3   Failure to Hold Justified Beliefs about Stressors Undermines Autonomy in Depression

The significance of the preceding discussion for autonomy in depression can now be detailed. There is a widespread but largely unjustified belief among sufferers that depression is a primary brain disorder. This view is reinforced by a dominant medical paradigm that supports a biological or brain-based conception of depression. There is also evidence that the biological model is further inculcated by high rates of ADM prescription. Put simply, many embrace the seemingly rational inference that if a treatment that directly targets brain chemistry is warranted, the underlying medical problem is caused by a primary derangement of neurochemistry. It also seems that, for many, brain-based and psychosocial conceptions of depression exist in competition, so that as the biological model gains prominence, appreciation of the role of stressors lessens. I have argued that an understanding of stressors is material to depressed people. I base this on the claim that for a stressor to trigger a depressive episode, it has been appraised as taxing and thus highly relevant to the depressed person's interests. Accurate information about the stressor–depression relationship is material because it is integral to addressing the stressor's causes, effects, and solutions, as well as the resulting depression. A failure to hold justified beliefs about this material relationship undermines, therefore, the autonomy with which the depressed person deals with the stressor and with his or her own depression.

Consider, for example, a depressed person in a situation of financial hardship, with a dependent family and a large mortgage. That person faces an array of decisions pertaining to the management of both finances and depression. These will likely include, "Should I refinance and seek a lower interest loan?," "Is this mortgage sustainable in the longer term, and, if not, ought we to sell the house and buy something more affordable?," "Should we make expenditure cuts, and, if so, what areas of our budget should we rein in?," "Ought I to seek a promotion to a higher paid but more stressful position in my organization?," "What kinds of activities should I engage in or avoid to hasten recovery from depression, and to avert recurrences?," and so on. It is plausible that the person who understands the stressor–depression link might reframe each of these questions with the prefix, "*Given my financial issues very likely comprise a stressor triggering a potentially life-threatening illness, depression, should I...*" One can imagine a range of possible responses that incorporate this information, including, "Finances are seriously stressful for me. I should delegate these tasks, and perhaps it would be worth hiring an accountant," "If our present mortgage is a source of ongoing stress, for the sake of my health it might be prudent to seek cheaper accommodation," "Budget cuts are unpleasant, but the knowledge they may lessen my depression risk will motivate my family to adapt," and "If my depression is stressor-related, perhaps a work promotion should be avoided at this time, despite the attractive remuneration." The addition of this material information contributes to autonomous choice with its associated value, including the protection of interests and enhanced control during a threatening state of affairs. Conversely, a failure to prefix these kinds of decisions with material understanding seriously undercuts the individual's prospects of exercising substantial autonomy in these areas.

This effect is exacerbated by a negative attributional style which, even when stressors are identified, works to distort their appraisal. In the current example, negative cognitive style could conceivably lead to the following skewed appraisals: "My money troubles have happened because I'm such a loser. My ineptitude obviously means similar catastrophes at work and in my personal relationships. I'm not sure I can face a future which offers only ongoing misery." Again, these are cognitions that can be informed by a prefix, for example, *"In a depressed state, I am more likely to blame myself excessively and to catastrophize the range and duration of outcomes..."* Given the materiality of information about the stressor–depression relationship, this prefix, and the broader understanding of cognitive biases to which it pertains, is integral to autonomous dealings with the stressor. It is plausible that its addition could alter responses in the following way: "Remember, there is a tendency in depression to overstate your responsibility for negative outcomes. Perhaps, rather than engaging in self-blame, it would be better to look at how these finances can be better managed," "It's easy when depressed to generalize bad outcomes to other areas and to the future. But my work and relationships are not the problem here. Financial issues are the key, so focus on those instead." These responses may seem improbably rational for someone with depression. However, in chapters 5 and 6, I will show how this kind of approach is feasible and can lead to more accurate stressor appraisals. Responses that omit this understanding demonstrate diminished autonomy, heightened risk to interests, and lessened effective control.

Because negative attributional style is, at least in part, mediated by negative affect, it is possible to extend to it the argument from the preceding chapter. There, I proposed that negative affect in depression has low evidential value in that it can strengthen the conviction with which unjustified beliefs are held about the affective trigger. I have demonstrated here that negative affect works to reinforce unjustified negative attributions. A failure to understand that negative affect engenders improbable assignations of self-blame and unduly dire judgments about the range and severity of outcomes militates against a realistic appreciation of the role of stressors. Given the materiality of facts concerning stressors, a failure to hold justified beliefs about depressed affect, and how it skews judgment, diminishes the autonomy of related decisions in depression.

To summarize, there is a strong case that negative information-processing biases distort the depressed person's worldview. Moreover, because depression is often triggered by stressors whose effective management is pivotal to the individual's interests, accurate perception and appraisal becomes a material matter. Failure to identify affect in depression as having poor evidential value, and a blinkered acceptance of the erroneous cognitions to which it gives rise, leads to decisions whose autonomy is frustrated by ignorance of material information. Thwarted autonomy augurs poorly for the individual's prominent interests and for his or her chances of exercising control in adverse situations. These observations make starkly clear that more is at stake in the treatment of depression than symptom relief, important though that goal may be. Choice of treatment carries profound implications for the autonomy impairment that stalks those with depression. In the subsequent two chapters I detail how CBT can help the depressed person understand his or her affective response in relation to both negative biases and the role of stressors. As a consequence, I will argue, CBT preserves and promotes the autonomy of the depressed person in a manner and to an extent that treatment with antidepressant medication alone cannot.

5 Understanding Negative Biases Promotes Autonomy in Depression

In the previous chapter, I argued that a number of factors conspire against the exercise of autonomy by people with depression. I showed that negative biases breed a pessimism, with doubtful warrant, that pervades judgments about important life events. I also argued biological beliefs about depression causation to be prominent in Western society, likely resulting from a dominant medical view that depression is "brain based," in concert with the widespread prescription of ADM. I showed such beliefs to be, in the main, unjustified and to work against the material understanding of psychosocial stressors as causal in depression. I also argued that, even when stressors are identified, negative attributional style can thwart their accurate appraisal. I concluded that a primary source of the autonomy impairment in depression is a failure to hold justified beliefs about the poor evidential value of affect. An understanding that depressed affect skews appraisals is a prerequisite for the systematic evaluation of triggering life events. It is this kind of empirical analysis that is most likely to lead to justified beliefs about material facts in the setting of a worldview that is permeated with negative affective bias. Now, I want to determine how autonomy impairment in depression is addressed by its two principal, validated treatments, CBT and ADM. In the current chapter, I investigate how each treatment deals with negative information-processing biases, and in the next chapter I focus on how each addresses the psychosocial stressors that can trigger depression.

CBT and ADM both counter negative biases, but two differences in the way these treatments "debias" depressive pessimism permit a moral demarcation between them. First, CBT requires the depressed individual to *understand* the action of negative biases. Through mindfulness, and the related skill metacognitive awareness, cognitions primed by negative affect are viewed with detached skepticism until confirmed or refuted by empirical investigation. A prerequisite of this approach is acceptance of the poor evidential value of negative affect in depression. The therapeutic effect of ADM requires no similar kind of comprehension. Given the materiality of justified beliefs about the poor evidence afforded by depressed affect, I argue that CBT confers a prima facie autonomy advantage. However, there is a second point of difference, which derives from evidence suggesting ADM limits the amplitude of negative affective swings. I argue that negative affect retains some utility, even in depression, to mark events of material significance. Despite depression's status as a disorder, its constituent affect has a residual appraisal function. The depressed person treated with ADM is, therefore, constrained in using negative affect to flag occurrences relevant to his or her interests. I argue that the CBT-treated person can, through negative affect, better identify significant events and more accurately assess them. As a result, he or she is well placed to hold justified beliefs about material facts concerning triggering events. These effects, taken together, suggest that CBT promotes the autonomy of the depressed person, not just in a different way, but also to a greater extent, than does treatment with ADM alone. To mount the argument, it is first necessary to understand what is known of the therapeutic mechanism of CBT in depression.

5.1 Mode of Action of Psychotherapy in Depression

In a widely cited definition, Hans Strupp has proposed the psychotherapeutic intervention to be

[a]n interpersonal process designed to bring about modifications of feelings, cognitions, attitudes and behaviour which have proved troublesome to the person seeking help from a trained professional.[1]

Of more than four hundred types of psychotherapy identified,[2] only a handful has been shown to benefit depression in controlled trials. The most extensively evaluated and clearly substantiated is CBT,[3] which, I will show, is an exemplar of Strupp's definition. Other therapies that have been subject to clinical trials, with generally favorable results, include mindfulness-based cognitive therapy (MBCT)[4], IPT,[5] and problem-solving therapy.[6] While these treatments will not be considered in detail, the autonomy claims I make for CBT would also apply to them, should they achieve benchmark efficacy and afford the kind of knowledge I hold to be material in depression.

In the previous chapter, I described the relationship between affect and cognition in depression as one of "mutual reinforcement." If I augur unpleasantness, negative affect convinces me that my gloomy outlook is accurate. Conversely, when unhappy, I take my negative thoughts as warrant for those feelings. However, it is important to appreciate that much of the relationship between affect and cognition in depression exists outside of awareness. The cognitive theory proposes a plausible framework with which to conceptualize this relationship. Negative thoughts are frequently "automatic," occurring effortlessly and spontaneously in the setting of triggering circumstances.[7] These so-called "negative automatic thoughts" are often self-referential, with the individual labeling himself or herself as a primary cause of negative outcomes. On one view, negative automatic thoughts foment lowered mood, which, in turn, through mood-congruent processing, sets off further negative cognitions. It is also possible that lowered mood is the prime mover and that, consistent with the "mood state" hypothesis described in the previous chapter, negative automatic thoughts appear consequent to dysphoria.[8] In either case, on the cognitive theory, there is activation of "dysfunctional attitudes" that form part of an individual's schematic way of viewing the world.[9] In chapter 4, "schema" was explained as an ingrained mode of responding to circumstances that derives from a person's unique set of experiences. Schemata typically become active during an experience of stress. Under the influence of schema, negative automatic thoughts are consolidated as "cognitive distortions" embodying a misshapen perspective of events.[10] This relationship is represented in figure 5.1.

It is instructive to apply this framework to the case of Penelope, considered in the previous chapter. Penelope is apparently snubbed by Harriet, a situation that triggers the automatic thought "Harriet is ignoring me

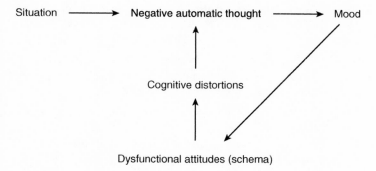

Figure 5.1
Cognitive model of depressive episode causation.

because she doesn't like me." This conclusion is reached instantaneously without any weighing of considerations. The negative thought catalyzes depressed mood and the activation of schemata and dysfunctional attitudes. A typical dysfunctional attitude is a sense of worthlessness or inadequacy. In Penelope's case, the resulting cognitive distortion might be "Of course Harriet doesn't like me—no one does, because I'm a loser." Were Penelope to seek help from a health professional trained in CBT, evidence for a diagnosis of depression would be sought according to *DSM-IV-TR* criteria.[11] She might have a history of lowered mood, poor concentration, difficulty making decisions, disrupted sleep, and reduced appetite. There could be increased fatigue and greater effort required to perform normal activities. She might also feel ashamed and inadequate when interacting socially. Intervention would focus on current triggers for lowered mood but would ultimately seek to locate those triggers within Penelope's core self-beliefs, beliefs molded by her idiosyncratic personal history.

Penelope and her therapist would engage in "collaborative empiricism" to establish the veracity of depressed cognitions.[12] The therapist would seek alternative explanations for Harriet's behavior, a process flagged in the discussion of this scenario in the previous chapter. Could Harriet be distracted by a work project or a personal issue? Is she under stress at the moment, and, if so, might that explain her behavior? If Harriet were just preoccupied, how likely is it that her actions were borne of disapproval or disdain? This technique might lead to "reattribution," with Penelope according greater weight to other possible interpretations of the encounter.[13] Dysfunctional attitudes and cognitive distortions would also be explored. Penelope has assumed that Harriet dislikes her and so labels herself a "loser." The therapist might question the logic of this inference. What, precisely, in the opinions of others constitutes evidence of her inadequacies? Do her spouse and friends also see her as a loser? If they do not, why should the opinion of one person justify such a conclusion? Why does the view of one person define her so totally while the views of her loved ones seem not to count? And so on. When negative cognitions with a tenuous factual basis are countered, depressed mood can lift.

It must be emphasized that, to date, no study has established with certainty the precise mechanism by which CBT exerts its therapeutic effect. However, it is a central claim of the cognitive theory that correction of cognitive errors is elemental to alleviation of depressive symptoms through CBT. Given the evidence that biased information processing mediates cognitive distortions in depression, it is reasonable to infer that renunciation of those cognitions after empirical challenge comprises a "debiasing" effect. Further if cognitive change is truly causal in symptom relief in depression, debiasing is a strong candidate for the responsible mechanism. Hayes and Hesketh mooted this relationship over two decades ago,[14] but research has been slow to substantiate this view. A primary difficulty has been to establish the causal direction between cognitions and depression.[15] Are more positive cognitions a nonspecific accompaniment of a depression that remits for other reasons? Or, does depression remit and recover as a result of more positive cognitions? I want to present some data that support the latter case and, therefore, debiasing as an active phenomenon in CBT. However, my primary goal is not to prove irrefutably that the effectiveness of CBT is mediated by cognitive change. Rather, I aim merely to show that CBT *involves* the understanding of negative biases and their correction through a range of techniques. Even though my argument will suggest this to be causal in successful CBT, it does not depend on proving such causation, for it is understanding the confounding nature of cognitions generated through negative affect that is central to the autonomy gains proposed here through psychotherapy. The argument remains intact whether that understanding causes or merely accompanies depressive symptom relief.

5.1.1 Evidence for Debiasing in CBT

The cognitive arm of CBT is thought to exert its effect by increasing the representation of more positive data in the depressed person's calculations, countering negative biases. In order to construe this as a debiasing effect, it is illustrative to consider a range of data suggesting debiasing, both outside and within a mental health context, to be a robust phenomenon.

Hirt and Markman have evaluated the "Consider an alternative" debiasing technique.[16] They asked study participants to read a hypothetical description of the work practices of firefighters, who were labeled either "risky" or "conservative," depending on how they carried out their duties. Subjects were then presented with data on the success rates of individual firefighters and whether they took a "risky" or a "conservative" approach to their job.[17] Participants were later divided into two groups, which were both asked to provide explanations for possible correlations between a risky approach and success as a firefighter. Explanations were sought for a positive, a negative, or an absent correlation between riskiness and success. The second group was subsequently required to give an additional explanation that differed from the first. Thus, in the second group, a participant initially asked to explain a positive correlation between riskiness and success might later be asked to explain a negative correlation. Both groups were also asked to rate their *actual* assessment of the correlation between riskiness and success as a firefighter at the end of each explanation task.

The investigators hypothesized that subjects would demonstrate an "explanation bias," which posits that outcomes will be deemed more probable if they are easier to explain.[18] It might be recalled, from chapter 4, that MacLeod and colleagues found evidence for an explanation bias in depression.[19] Thus, depressed people were more able to generate explanations for negative outcomes and also judged those outcomes to be more likely, supporting a link between explanation accessibility and subjective probability. Like MacLeod and colleagues, Hirt and Markman believe the explanation bias is underpinned by the availability heuristic or by its extension, simulation. The availability heuristic was explained in chapter 4 as the propensity for individuals to "assess the frequency of a class or the probability of an event by the ease with which instances or occurrences can be brought to mind."[20] Simulation proposes that the probability of future events is assessed by the ease with which a mental simulation of those events can be made.[21] Accepting this account, ready explanation might bias probability assessments because the explained outcomes are easier to mentally access, or to simulate.

The study was supportive of the researchers' hypothesis. Subjects required to explain a particular risk–success correlation were more likely to believe that such a correlation actually held. Thus, those explaining a positive correlation between riskiness and success were more likely to accept it, rather than a negative correlation, as factual. However, it is the investigators' next finding that most strongly supports debiasing as an active phenomenon; they found an effect to *reverse* the initial explanation bias in the second group, who were asked to give additional, countering explanations. Thus, those who first explained a positive correlation and then had to explain a negative correlation gave a more negative rating of the actual correlation after the second task. The investigators propose that debiasing alters likelihood assessments by increasing the availability, or ease of simulation, of alternative explanations.

Specific support for debiasing as a therapeutic mechanism in the mental health arena comes from Bentz and colleagues. They studied individuals with and without anxiety undergoing a "Consider an alternative" debiasing procedure.[22] In this study, subjects were asked to rate the likelihood of various threat-related events and scenarios. For example:

You are late for an important meeting across town so you are driving above the speed limit. It starts to rain heavily and the traffic around you is hard to see clearly. What is the probability that you will have/will avoid a car accident?[23]

Anxious subjects were significantly more likely to predict adverse outcomes than were nonanxious subjects. Later, all participants underwent a debiasing procedure, which involved generating three alternative, positive outcomes for the target events. For example, in the first scenario, an alternative outcome might involve pulling the car over, turning off the engine, and ringing the meeting convener to convey what has happened. When likelihood ratings were repeated after debiasing, there was a significant reduction in pessimistic predictions in both groups.

Evidence of debiasing during CBT is also suggested by data supporting cognitive change as a mediator of therapeutic effect in depression. Around 40 percent of depressed patients experience more than half of their total symptom improvement during one interval between therapy sessions.[24] These rapid improvements, termed "sudden gains," are predictive of improved outcomes, in particular, lower relapse rates.[25] Importantly, the gains seem to occur independent of life events and are associated with specific cognitive changes. Such changes include identifying errors in cognitive processes or beliefs, arriving at a new schema, recognizing errors in an existing schema, and accepting a new cognitive technique. [26] For example, one participant, on relinquishing a belief that she was unattractive because her boyfriend had left her, stated, "I can't believe I actually thought that! How could I let him decide if I am attractive or not?"[27] Investigators categorized this as identification of an error in a cognitive process. Sudden gains describe alterations in depressed cognitions that likely result from empirical challenge through CBT, a process consistent with the debiasing techniques considered. The data implicating sudden gains as predictive of superior symptom relief in depression are, therefore, suggestive that debiasing may operate in CBT.

Consideration of actual case studies, and the prominence of alternative interpretations of events, lends intuitive weight to debiasing as an active element of CBT. The following example, involving a 51-year-old bank manager with moderate depression, is representative:

Client: I can't tell you how much of a mess I've made of things. I've made another major error of judgment, which should cost me my job.
Therapist: Tell me what the error in judgment was.
C: I approved a loan, which fell through completely. I made a very poor decision.

T: Can you recall the specifics about the decision?

C: Yes, I remember that it looked good on paper, good collateral, good credit rating, but I should have known there was going to be a problem.

T: Did he have all the pertinent information at the time of your decision?

C: Not at the time, but I sure found out six weeks later. I'm paid to make profitable decisions, not to give the bank's money away.

T: I understand your position, but I would like to review the information which you had at the time your decision was required, not six weeks after the decision had been made.[28]

The authors then describe what followed:

When the therapist and patient reviewed the pertinent information available at the time of his decision, the patient reasonably concluded that his initial decision was based on sound banking principles. He even recalled checking the client's financial background intensively.[29]

The banker's initial construal displays a negative attributional style. As discussed in the previous chapter, negative attributions are well explained by the biased information processing that takes place in depression. A stressor, in this case a loan default, is not viewed as possessing inherently taxing properties. Rather, the banker assigns the entire responsibility for the adverse outcome to his own behavior. Consideration of plausible alternative factors contributing to the unfavorable result counters the excessive weight placed on the banker's own actions as causal. While the resulting reattribution does not divest the banker of all blame, it does embody a more realistic distribution of responsibility to the parties involved. It coheres with the mechanisms discussed that reattribution of responsibility results from a debiasing of negative attributions through the consideration of alternative explanations.

     The mechanism of action of CBT proposed by John Teasdale and colleagues is also consistent with a debiasing effect.[30] They use the analogy of word stems. For example, when asked to complete the stem MOU_ _, most will do so with the more common word MOUSE rather than the less common MOUND. This would appear to be a straightforward application of the availability heuristic. If someone uses the word MOUSE frequently, it follows that it will be more readily brought to mind than a term employed less often. Teasdale and colleagues note that exposing subjects to prior presentations of the word MOUND can reverse this tendency, an effect consistent with a debiasing of availability through increasing the accessibility of alternative word endings. Teasdale extends the analogy to the schemata that feature in depressive episodes, suggesting that part of the effect of CBT is to provide alternative "endings" to the scenarios that generally trigger depression. As a result, more positive and realistic conclusions become increasingly available for information processing. For example, the depressed bank manager typically responds to stressors with feelings of ineptitude and assignations of self-blame, but serial challenge lessens the frequency of this mode of response. As Teasdale puts it:

[CBT] leads to repeated experiences in which alternative, less depressogenic, schematic models concerning depression, its symptoms and effects, and related problematic life situations, are synthesised and stored in memory.[31]

Teasdale goes on to explain that access to more adaptive responses to depressive triggers will likely depend on the presence, in memory, of

many episodic representations of the more adaptive patterns in conjunction with a wide variety of contexts. These representations, in turn, will have to be created on many occasions, in many different contexts, if they, rather than depressogenic representations, are to be accessed.[32]

Thus, on this model, schemata might be ingrained but they are not immutable. A process like debiasing can gradually construct a schematic model that differs from the one the individual is used to. This process is facilitated by two further techniques: metacognitive awareness and behavioral strategies.

5.1.2 Metacognitive Awareness and Mindfulness

Teasdale is also a proponent of strategies, often combined with CBT, to help the depressed person gain *metacognitive awareness*, which, as outlined in the previous chapter, describes a distanced or decentered perspective in relation to negative feelings and thoughts.[33] Rather than submitting to an uncritical and often automatic response to negative moods and cognitions, metacognitive awareness involves identifying these "mental events" as not always indicative of reality. Thoughts are not engaged with but rather "let go," which, combined with skepticism about their validity, can interrupt rumination and the progression to depression.[34] Mindfulness, also discussed in the previous chapter, is a meditative and philosophical approach that assists in attaining metacognitive awareness. Allen and colleagues provide a helpful definition:

Mindfulness involves "paying attention in a particular way: on purpose, in the present moment, and non-judgementally."[35] It refers to the cultivation of conscious awareness and attention on a moment-to-moment basis. The quality of awareness sought by mindfulness practice includes openness or receptiveness, curiosity and a non-judgmental attitude. An emphasis is placed on seeing and accepting things as they are without trying to change them. Mindfulness is contrasted with habitual mental functioning or "being on automatic pilot."[36]

The meditative aspect of mindfulness emphasizes a conscious focus on the breath that is maintained even when thoughts intrude and vie for attention. Thoughts that persistently incur are not ushered away or suppressed but simply "watched." Metacognitive awareness and mindfulness have been shown to be effective in preventing depressive relapse.[37] These approaches require an understanding that negative thoughts and mood confound expectations of the utility of actions and so reinforce wariness about taking depressed cognitions and affect as guides to behavior.

5.1.3   Behavioral Aspects of CBT

Depressed people are less motivated to do things that were once pleasurable. In part, this relates to the enervation of depression, but there is also a perception that goals are either unachievable or will not be enjoyed. The aim of behavioral intervention is to provide experiential evidence to the contrary.[38] When a depressed person succeeds where he or she anticipated failure, evidence is adduced for ability, rather than incompetence. If a dreaded outing is actually enjoyed, the possibility of agreeable experience becomes tangible. In the terminology of CBT, these activities are evidence of "mastery" and "pleasure" which can alter negative self-assessments.[39] The outcomes indicate ability to achieve satisfaction and can motivate behavior—such as accepting invitations rather than staying home—that reinforce positive cognitions.

The preceding discussion indicates that an understanding of the action of negative biases is a central outcome of successful CBT. Acknowledging the role played by negative biases is a precondition to the generation of alternative interpretations of the causes and outcomes of aversive experiences. It is likely that consideration of differing explanations from those favored as part of the depressive response contributes to more realistic appraisals and the amelioration of depression. This technique may work by reversing mood-congruent biases that foster preferential inclusion of negative material in the thought processes of people with depression. Debiasing increases the availability of more positive renderings of distressing circumstances, heightening the chances that conclusions will take these alternative readings into account. If the individual is to successfully challenge depressive thoughts, it is advantageous to adopt a distanced and skeptical metacognitve standpoint when negative cognitions arise in the setting of lowered mood. Mindfulness is an approach that has been shown to facilitate such a stance and also to reduce risk of depressive relapse. While cognitive change has not been shown to be definitively causal in the therapeutic effect of CBT, the evidence is suggestive. For example, Hollon and DeRubeis recently concluded a review of studies assessing the role of cognitive mediation of symptom relief by stating the following:

Collectively, these studies suggest that patients' recognition of the role of cognition in depression and the growth of skills with respect to examining the accuracy of one's beliefs play a role in reducing risk for subsequent relapse.[40]

Yet, as explained earlier, while it is probable that cognitive change contributes to the therapeutic efficacy of CBT, it is not essential for the argument that follows to show such a connection to conclusively hold. For the argument at hand, it is the contribution of cognitive change to personal autonomy that has greatest relevance.

5.2 How CBT Promotes Autonomy in Depression; Understanding Biases

It is worthwhile reiterating why justified beliefs about affect are important for autonomy. Affect arises when a target event carries material significance for the agent. Affect provides evidence for the truth of associated propositions and for the value to the individual of the outcome of triggering encounters. However, the evidence of affect varies in quality, and so affect-driven determinations can be veridical or they can be false. If affect signifies materiality, the evidence afforded by it ought also to be viewed as material. It is important for autonomy that the agent holds justified beliefs about material facts and, therefore, about the evidence of affect. In chapter 4, I argued that mood-congruent biases in depression fuel unrealistic pessimism and that depressed affect has poor evidential value in that it tends to reinforce unjustified associated beliefs. Depressed people are poorly placed to see this and frequently treat negative affect as good evidence for their pessimistic forecasts. In short, those with depression often fail to hold justified beliefs about the evidential value of negative affect.

Much of CBT is devoted to informing the depressed person of the confounding nature of strong negative affect. Negative cognitions are challenged and often disowned. Erroneous conclusions drawn by the person with depression are brought out. Prima facie, apprising a person with depression of this material information ought to go some way to furthering his or her autonomy. Yet, merely supplying information, which may then be understood, can still fall short of the beliefs that are necessary for autonomy in depression. Depressive pessimism can be phenomenologically compelling and difficult to resist, even in the presence of solid countering evidence. It is plausible that a pervasive action of depressed affect to reinforce negative cognitions contributes. For example, the bank manager, discussed earlier, might acknowledge that the available information supported a loan approval and accept that he was largely blameless for the unfortunate turn of events. Nevertheless, a credible response might still be, "I was probably warranted in granting the loan. But I *feel* so bad; I *know* I must have done something wrong. Why else would I feel this way?"

I want to suggest three reasons why persistent negative affect could make it difficult for individuals to repudiate their pessimistic cognitions. First, extant depressed affect will continue to exert a mood-congruent bias and so negative construals will be accorded disproportionate weight in the agent's calculations. This mechanism might sustain pessimism in the face of contradicting empirical data. Second, as the Iowa Gambling Task and related research suggest, affect probably influences utility assessments and decision making outside of awareness. It is plausible, then, that unconscious affective input could make negative cognitions relatively immune to conscious manipulation. Finally, as discussed in chapter 3, we may be hardwired to err on the side of accepting our negative affective beliefs because, from an evolutionary perspective, it makes adaptive sense to maintain focus on threat. Each of these factors suggests it may be counterintuitive and difficult for depressed people to challenge the foreboding that accompanies negative affect.

These observations emphasize the importance for autonomy of the shift from taking depressed affect at face value, to viewing it with detachment. This is a prominent element of CBT and is facilitated by the depressed person's adopting a particular set of beliefs in relation to his or her affective response. For example, "Thoughts do not always indicate reality. Feelings do not always corroborate accompanying thoughts." Such beliefs underpin the resistance to engagement with negative cognitions that permits their interrogation and the renunciation of those that prove unfounded. In short, justified beliefs about the evidential value of affect lead to decisions with a firmer basis in fact and greater autonomy. Consider, for example, what might follow should the bank manager forgo therapy and base decisions on the view that his actions "should cost me my job." He could lose confidence in his judgment, become excessively cautious, and begin to withhold loans that had good reason to be granted. He could turn to alcohol or other drugs to deal with his fear of being dismissed. Alternatively, he might conceal details of the loan from other staff or from his superiors. In fact, the latter is precisely what happened in the case study reported by Beck and colleagues.[41] The banker avoided contacting the central office, which delayed the commencement of legal proceedings against the loan defaulter. This action was premised on self-blame, engendered by negative affect, and shown later to be unwarranted. Skepticism of conclusions made during periods of negative affect leads to more realistic appraisals of events and to related decisions that are more autonomous.

My contention is that the promotion of autonomy through CBT is greater than that achieved through the use of ADM alone. In order to substantiate this claim, it is necessary to look more closely at the mode of action of ADM in depression.

5.3   Mode of Action of Antidepressant Medication in Depression

A great deal is known about the effects of ADM on brain chemistry. The actions of ADM on serotonin, dopamine, noradrenaline, and downstream mediators such as BDNF have been extensively investigated.[42] Yet, surprisingly little is known of the neuropsychological mechanisms through which ADM exerts its therapeutic effect. In fact Catherine Harmer, an experimental psychologist at Oxford University, has made the following comment on the effects of ADM on brain chemistry: "[T]here is *no* neuropsychological account of how these changes relieve depressive states."[43]

Harmer herself appears to be one of few researchers working in this area. In a seminal study, her group administered citalopram, reboxetine (antidepressants acting on serotonin and noradrenaline, respectively), or placebo to healthy volunteers.[44] Participants were then tested on their perception of negative and positive emotional stimuli. First, they were shown pictures of human faces expressing happiness, surprise, sadness, fear, anger, and disgust.[45] The ADM-treated group was less able to recognize fearful and angry expressions compared to the placebo group. In addition, those in the citalopram group were significantly more likely to misclassify the three negative emotions—fear, anger, and disgust—as happiness. The findings supported the investigators' hypothesis that ADM promotes increased recognition of positive expressions and reduced recognition of negative expressions.

In a second task, emotional categorization, subjects were presented with 60 personality characteristics, each appearing on a screen for half a second.

Some characteristics were chosen to be disagreeable, such as dominance, hostility, and untidiness. Others were more agreeable, for example, cheerfulness, honesty, and optimism. Subjects were asked to rate characteristics as likeable or not likeable. The reboxetine group was significantly faster at categorizing agreeable traits as likeable than the placebo group, a finding also consistent with biased processing of positively valenced emotional stimuli. Immediately after emotional categorization, participants were asked to recall as many personality descriptions as possible from that task. In this test of "emotional memory," the total number of recalled words did not differ between the three groups. However, the ADM-treated groups recalled more positive words than did the placebo group. The authors concluded that ADM works to

reduce the processing of negative emotional material and increase memory for positively valenced items in healthy non-depressed volunteers. Such actions of antidepressants may act to reverse the pervasive negative biases in memory and information processing that are apparent during periods of clinical anxiety and depression.[46]

While the results of this study broadly replicated those of a similar study by the same group,[47] both experiments were limited by a failure to include participants with depression. Harmer's group addressed this limitation in a placebo controlled trial comparing the effects of reboxetine on patients with newly diagnosed, unmedicated depression against a control group of healthy volunteers.[48] Participants were administered the same battery of tests just described. Compared to controls, depressed patients who received placebo demonstrated reduced recognition of positive facial expressions, took longer to identify agreeable personality traits, and had poorer recall of those traits. These effects were reversed in depressed participants receiving reboxetine, with the increase in positive processing being similar to or larger than that seen in ADM-treated healthy controls, depending on the task. This study further suggests that ADM works to reverse negative affective biases in depression, and it supports the validity of the earlier studies that did not include a depressed cohort.

However, there is a particular finding in this study that must be considered in the argument to come. The researchers noted that when positive information processing increased, it did so independent of changes in measures of mood or anxiety. This finding is understandable considering the typical delay of some weeks between commencement of SSRI treatment and alleviation of depressive symptoms, and given that testing in the study was performed a mere 3 hours after drug administration. Nonetheless, the authors base a significant claim on this observation. They suggest that, when depression is treated with ADM, mood improvement is preceded by an automatic, pharmacologically induced correction of negative biases. In corroboration, the investigators cite a study showing that improved recognition of happy facial expressions after a week's administration of Citalopram predicts an eventual therapeutic response in depressed patients at 6 weeks.[49] Harmer and colleagues adduce these data as evidence for what they term a "cognitive neuropsychological model" of ADM action.[50] On this view, the time lag to depressive symptom relief with ADM accommodates a necessary cascade of effects between the very early reversal of negative biases and the later lifting of mood. That cascade, according to the authors, includes more positive environmental appraisals leading to responses, such as reduced social withdrawal, that subsequently reinforce upward shifts in mood. It is proposed that the nature and implications of social cues must be "relearned" by the depressed person undergoing ADM treatment, a process whose gradual time frame sets a template for the period over which mood improvement takes place. Thus, "changes in affective bias with antidepressant drug administration do not directly enhance mood, but may provide a platform for subsequent cognitive and psychological reconsolidation."[51]

These findings have significance for the argument to come in that they describe ADM exerting neuropsychological effects with very strong parallels to those proposed to mediate the effects of CBT. Thus, both treatments would seem to target the mood-congruent processing biases that characterize depressed thinking. If the two treatments share such an important therapeutic mechanism, one that relates so closely to the autonomy argument propounded, how is it possible to differentiate between their respective effects on autonomy in depression?

5.4   Comparing the Effects of CBT and ADM on Autonomy in Depression

The findings of Harmer's group raise an important question: if CBT augments autonomy through the reduction of mood-congruent biases, and ADM also reduces those biases, might ADM promote autonomy in depression in a similar way, and to a similar extent, as CBT? Grant, for the sake of argument, that the tendency of ADM to cause misclassification of some negative emotional stimuli is limited to healthy people, such as those in Harmer's earlier study. Thus, I'll accept, for the moment, that such obvious mistakes do not manifest in depressed individuals taking these medications. It seems that affect in depressed people taking ADM might regain the evidential value it had before depression emerged. If ADM reverses negative biases, then the resulting affect ought to reinforce veridical beliefs with a similar frequency to healthy affect. Further, there seems little reason for individuals to be any more or less skeptical of the evidential value of their drug-treated affect than of their predepression affect. Therefore, the justifiability of any beliefs they might hold in relation to their drug-treated affect ought to parallel that of their nondepressed state. Accepting this contention, and given the importance of justified beliefs about affect for autonomy, ADM appears to have the potential to return autonomy to predepression status. How, then, can the argument that CBT provides an autonomy advantage be sustained?

First, it should be noted that conclusions influenced by negative biases *prior* to drug treatment might still hold for the individual. Reconsider the case of depressed Penelope apparently shunned by work colleague Harriet. Her negatively biased assessment of that incident will not necessarily be "corrected" through later ADM administration. The influence of negative affect to prime a potentially false interpretation could plausibly persist. Even if free of negative bias in relation to extant and future circumstances, biased perceptions of past incidents, which occurred during a depressive episode, might remain. Here the acquisition of knowledge that comes through successful CBT can profit its holder. Through understanding the misleading properties of depressed affect, the CBT recipient can bring "collaborative empiricism" to bear on depressive instances that precede the treatment period. In this way, accurate evaluations can be made over broad periods that have been subject to the confounding influence of depression. Here is an initial reason to see CBT as providing an autonomy advantage over ADM.

However, there is a more pronounced enhancement of autonomy seen with psychotherapy. Recall that the effects of negative biases in depression *tend* to result in erroneous pessimism. Biases are not wholly inaccurate but result in an overall shift toward predictions of negative outcomes. Although biases make it more likely that negative predictions will be false, some pessimistic assessments might, in fact, be realistic. CBT works not by *eradicating* negative biases but by assisting the depressed person to *understand* them. Through that, CBT encourages skepticism of pessimistic predictions, and their empirical investigation. In many cases, it is likely that evaluation will lead to an appropriate disowning of negative predictions and to an alteration of subsequent decision making to reflect the new viewpoint. However, it is quite possible that some pessimistic forecasts, made in the presence of negative affect, will have good grounds. Understanding of biases leads to a kind of "filter of skepticism" in relation to views formed under the influence of negative affect. While the initial response of the CBT-treated person to negative cognitions will be wary and dubious, it remains possible he or she will conclude them to be justified. Ultimately, it is skepticism and investigation that is most likely to give rise to justified beliefs about the evidence afforded by negative affect.

Fairly clearly, ADM does not work like this. While the precise neuropsychological effects of ADM remain uncertain, there is probably a wholesale shift toward a more positive interpretation of stimuli. The findings of Harmer and colleagues, in particular those relating to the ADM-treated group who misclassified fear, anger, and disgust for happiness, support the existence of such a shift and its potential inaccuracies.[52] Also, while the cited data suggest that reduction in negative biases might precede affective change in ADM-treated depression, it is consistent with this model that affect undergoes a similar quantum positive shift, albeit slightly delayed. The philosophical problem with such an affective shift relates to the materiality of circumstances that normally trigger affect. I have shown that affect tends to be elicited when an agent's interests are closely tied to unfolding events. For that reason, I argue that the evaluations made in relation to affective triggers tend to be material to the agent. The emergence of affect in response to a life event tags that event with material significance for its percipient. Thus, for Penelope, a negative affective response to the apparent shunning by Harriet implies their relationship is one of importance for her principal interests. Further, it means the facts of the encounter will be relevant to the fulfillment of those interests. If the episode truly represents shunning, then there are considerable implications for the future of, for example, their joint projects. The concern is that, if ADM behaves in the way presented, it may limit the capacity for affect to vary appropriately with the emotive content of environmental stimuli. As a result, a constraint is placed on the agent's ability to detect interest-relevant events and to mark them out as requiring systematic and focused evaluation. In the absence of this sense apparatus, there is no signal that a stimulus merits further inquiry to arrive at justified beliefs concerning its threat potential. If the opportunity to arrive at justified beliefs about a material occurrence is limited, autonomous responses are jeopardized, and associated interests placed at risk.

There is empirical evidence to support the kinds of affective shifts mooted here. In particular, there is evidence that the negative affective range of those taking ADM is constrained. Knutson and colleagues administered either the ADM paroxetine or placebo to never-depressed volunteers.[53] They found a significant reduction in the experience of negative affect in the ADM-treated group. Moreover, the extent to which negative affect decreased correlated with serum levels of the ADM. The investigators also conducted open-ended interviews at the conclusion of the study, asking, "What did you experience during the experiment." One subject responded, "I used to think about good and bad, but now I don't. I'm in a good mood," providing some qualitative affirmation of the study's conclusion.[54] Simmons and colleagues, in an unpublished study, administered the ADM fluoxetine or placebo to 40 healthy volunteers.[55] They found constrained mood in those receiving ADM, with a restriction in the amplitude of both positive and negative affect. Similar observations were made by Opbroek and colleagues, who assessed emotional responsiveness in a group of patients with remitted depression who were taking ADM and who had experienced medication-induced sexual dysfunction.[56] The investigators found that subjects, relative to controls, experienced significantly less ability to cry, feel sadness, or to care about the feelings of others, a result they termed "emotional blunting."[57] More recently, Price and colleagues conducted semistructured interviews in people taking SSRI ADM.[58] The majority of participants were medicated for depression, with a small number being treated for anxiety disorders. Most individuals reported a general reduction in the intensity of emotions, using adjectives such as "dulled," "numbed," and "flattened" to describe their feelings. Almost all participants experienced a reduction in the frequency and intensity of positive emotions, reporting these feelings as "dampened down," or "toned down." Unsurprisingly, all experienced a reduction in negative emotions such as sadness, anger, anxiety, worry, and fear. Of interest, though, some described this as an adverse effect. As the authors explained,

[a]lthough a reduction in these negative emotions was usually at some stage a benefit or relief, for many participants it had become an unwanted side-effect, impairing their quality of life. Participants described the need to be able to feel negative emotions when appropriate, such as grief or concern. Some were unable to respond with negative emotions, such as being able to cry when this would have been appropriate or respond appropriately to bad news.[59]

The actions of ADM in these studies lend weight to the following claim. The strength of CBT, against pharmacotherapy, is that the potential for affect to mark events as material is not ablated, or blunted in a way that renders it insensitive to the particulars of the situation. Affect can still "track" events and mark occurrences of significance. At the same time, it can be held at arm's length, in terms of its action-guiding utility, until evaluation corroborates or refutes interpretations fueled by it. In the process CBT engenders, I contend, justified beliefs about events of material significance to the individual. ADM does not seem to afford this opportunity. In shifting the affective spectrum to positive, ADM appears to reduce the potential of negative affect to arise as a marker of events tied to the individual's interests. Also, lacking skills with which to evaluate the implications of such events, those treated with ADM have a reduced capacity to arrive at justified beliefs about them.

In light of these data, it is instructive to reconsider the case of Penelope. Imagine she had been treated with ADM prior to the corridor incident. It is plausible that she is now less likely to experience negative affect on being, ostensibly, ignored by her colleague. Accepting the view that affect arises when interests are at issue, it is likely to be material to Penelope if Harriet is avoiding her. It might, for example, indicate their collaborative projects to be in jeopardy. Negative affect marks the event as warranting further evaluation, which will yield information that is important to guide decisions about continuation of their joint work. Now, if negative affect does not emerge from the encounter, perhaps as a result of medication, there seems a real chance that an event of material significance will be overlooked. There will be no trigger to evaluate the incident and to see if evidence bears out Penelope's interpretation. In short, there will be a reduced ability to achieve the most justified beliefs in relation to that event. If the goal is to identify, and to achieve justified appraisals of, material circumstances, it is better to perceive events with an intact affective range and to cognitively evaluate one's interpretation than to be limited in one's affective scope.[60] If such a process leads to more justified beliefs, it follows that, in those applying the skills of CBT, affect tends to track a more realistic construal of events. Affect, rather than being pharmacologically induced, occurs when an event is *understood* in a different and probably more accurate way. In CBT, positive affect arises when states of affairs are understood to be more favorable than was previously thought. Affect can retain its role as a marker of environmental events of significance and comprise a sign that threats to an agent's interests have been averted. Affect retains something of its role as a tool of appraisal.

This is not obviously the case with ADM, which can improve affect without any altered or improved understanding of events in the world. ADM-induced affect appears less likely to track states of affairs, measure potential threats to the agent's interests, or improve when such threats are vitiated. Affect engendered by ADM seems to come with a broadly positive take on the world. In light of the ADM effect to mitigate negative biases, such a view might be more realistic than that of the person with depression who remains untreated. However, the formerly depressed person, newly armed with the skills of CBT, seems better equipped to arrive at justified beliefs in relation to events of material significance to him or her. This is because some incidents *shouldn't* be seen more positively, for example, those that put goals at risk and therefore invite rectification. In Penelope's corridor encounter, if joint projects were truly under threat, it would be imprudent to disregard the incident.

In reply, it might be objected that many incidents that generate negative affective swings for the untreated depressive will not be material to his or her interests. The reasoning behind this objection is that the depressed person's propensity to impute threat or loss where there is none will lead to a greater number of incidents appraised as material, and warranting investigation, when there is no cause for concern. For example, it is known that depressed people are more likely to interpret facial expressions and comments in social contexts as self-referential, aversive, and unpleasant.[61] In addition, it is known that in depression there is hyperarousal of the amygdala,[62] a key brain region in the processing of threat cues, which may mediate this kind of negative information processing. Moreover, Harmer's group has found that never-depressed volunteers administered an SSRI ADM and exposed to threatening stimuli (fearful facial expressions) have reduced responsiveness of amygdala, hippocampus, and medial prefrontal cortex.[63] This finding is consistent with other data suggesting ADM acts directly to diminish amygdala activity in depression.[64] These data support the cognitive neuropsychological account, which proposes ADM to elevate mood indirectly through altered processing of threat-related, emotionally salient stimuli. So, ADM may not simply ramp up mood as a blunt neuro-chemical effect but, rather, attenuate the overvigilant monitoring of potential threat, with mood lifting as a consequence of that modified processing. If this account is accepted, the mood constraint, or limitation of affective swings, that seems to occur with ADM might be the *result* of diminished sensitivity to interest-*irrelevant* events, rather than the *cause* of diminished sensitivity to interest-*relevant* events. This construal suggests that the CBT-treated person who attends to and scrutinizes those incidents that generate negative affective swings might gain more justified beliefs about them, but because the incidents are immaterial such beliefs will have minimal bearing on his or her autonomy. ADM may not obliterate a useful affective response to threat but, perhaps by dampening an overactive amygdala, simply maintains that response at a manageable level unlikely to lead to depression. If this account is accurate, it raises the possibility that affect in the unmedicated depressive is too sensitive to be a useful marker of materiality and that affect in those treated with ADM might have greater utility in this regard.

A number of replies can be made to this potential objection. First, recall the misclassification as "happy" of fearful and angry expressions in the Harmer study cited earlier. While the preceding argument grants that drug development might reduce such inaccuracies, Harmer's finding suggests pharmacologists and clinicians will face major challenges calibrating ADM information processing to a level that permits accurate interpretation of potentially threatening events. This point is supported by the studies on mood constraint seen with SSRI use. If negative affect is limited such that, for example, individuals cannot feel appropriate sadness in response to distressing circumstances, it seems likely that the underlying bias correction has been excessive. By contrast, the "understanding" approach offered by CBT uses empirical interrogation as the ultimate barometer of threat acuity and so seems to provide a more "all weather" tool for threat appraisal. Thus, while a greater number of incidents may be subject to cognitive reappraisal with CBT, this technique makes it less likely that true threats will be overlooked. Moreover, even if calibration could be perfected so that affective responses to threat or loss in ADM-treated depression approximated those in healthy people, the everyday fallibility of emotional appraisal means that even here affectively driven conclusions might be mistaken. As a result, the cognitive evaluation advocated as a prudent accompaniment to most negative affective assessments will likely still prove advantageous in achieving the most accurate interpretation of events. Further, it must be remembered that depressed mood lifts with successful CBT, suggesting that, as treatment progresses, cognitive changes result in reduced "gain" in the amygdala response. Thus, it seems likely that unwarranted negative affect, and false positive marking of triggering events as material, will reduce as the disorder ameliorates. This claim is supported by early neuroimaging data suggesting that cognitive therapy might also normalize the amygdala hyperreactivity that occurs in depression.[65] DeRubeis and colleagues hypothesize that cognitive therapy recruits "top down" cortical pathways to dampen amygdala activity in depression, in contrast to ADM action, which targets the amygdala directly.[66] If this account proves accurate, it provides reason to think those who successfully undertake CBT may be no more prone to overdetermining instances of threat than those who receive ADM.

As a result, recalling the importance of justified beliefs in relation to material facts for autonomy, it remains my contention that CBT has a greater potential than ADM to augment the autonomy of decisions and actions made by the depressed individual in relation to negative affective triggers. Further, the depressed person's beliefs about the significance of his or her affective response play a prominent role in this process. In consequence, it is reasonable to hold that justified beliefs concerning the evidence of affect mediate the autonomy promotion seen in the depressed person successfully treated with CBT. In the next chapter, my task will be to examine how CBT and ADM address psychosocial stressors and consider the implications of their respective effects for the autonomy of the person with depression.

6   Understanding Causal Stressors Promotes Autonomy in Depression

I will now argue that psychotherapy promotes autonomy in depression by creating awareness of the causal role of psychosocial stressors and of effective means of dealing with them. I will further argue that the autonomy-promoting effects of CBT are superior to those of ADM. The argument hinges on the claim, defended in chapter 4, that a causal role for stressors will be material to those with depression. That claim had two primary grounds. First, their capacity to evoke negative affect signals stressors as threats to interests. Stressors threaten interests not simply by precipitating an unpleasant affective disorder but because depression itself hampers the individual setting things right in relation to the stressful event. Second, causal factors for illness are material to sufferers because their understanding affords additional options for dealing with the illness. The asthmatic aware of the deleterious effects of cigarette smoke, or the angina sufferer who understands the link between cholesterol and heart disease, gains knowledge of additional preventative measures. CBT, I will argue now, not only aims to elucidate causal stressors but also teaches strategies to manage them. In this way, CBT can protect important interests, and so the knowledge it affords, I argue, is material to those with depression. I show that ADM can also, theoretically, promote the autonomy of the depressed person's response to stressful life events. However, I conclude that because ADM does not impart material understanding, it promotes autonomy in depression in a different way and to a lesser extent than does CBT. To build my case, it is first necessary to clarify how CBT addresses the psychosocial stressors that trigger depression.

6.1   Mode of Action of CBT in Depression; Addressing Stressors

In chapter 5, I outlined how CBT could ameliorate depression by promoting awareness of information-processing biases. This facet of psychotherapy can be construed as targeting the "diathesis" element in the "stress–diathesis" model of depression causation. Here, diathesis refers to the individual's tendency to perceive and process stimuli in a way that renders him or her vulnerable to a depressive response. However, CBT also aims to elucidate and address the stressful life events that are frequently implicated in depression. But to say that stressors exist on one side of a clear-cut, "stress–diathesis" divide would be an oversimplification. Although some life events, such as assault or marriage breakdown, are experienced as stressful by most people, vulnerable individuals evince stress at lower thresholds. Given a sufficiently sensitive diathesis even apparently trivial adversity can be perceived as stressful. Bruce McEwen, a respected researcher in the field, reflects this observation when he defines stress as "an event or events that are *interpreted* as threatening to an individual and which elicit physiological and behavioral responses."[1] In cases of heightened vulnerability, it is of manifest importance to address perceptual distortions mediated by information-processing biases. However, as I will explain later in this chapter, even in situations of excessive sensitivity, stressor-focused approaches can have benefit.

Several types of psychotherapy contain elements that specifically target stressors. For example, CBT, IPT,[2] problem-solving therapy,[3] and cognitive behavior stress management (CBSM)[4] all address situational factors contributing to the individual's distress. Of these, CBT[5] IPT,[6] and problem-solving therapy[7] have been shown, in controlled trials, to be effective in depression. CBSM warrants special mention as it has been demonstrated to prevent cortisol rises in response to stressful events. In chapter 4, I explained that stress-induced cortisol elevation is suspected to be an etiological factor in depression.[8] CBSM teaches a number of different strategies, including problem solving, which are common to CBT. In two studies evaluating CBSM, participants took the Trier Social Stress Test, which has been shown to elicit cortisol-mediated stress responses in healthy subjects.[9,10] The test requires completion of an arithmetic task and attending a simulated job interview in front of a small audience. After the test, those trained in CBSM had significantly lower cortisol elevations than controls with no CBSM training. Given the significance of cortisol responses in the genesis of depression, these findings suggest an important role for stressor-oriented therapies in its treatment.

The stressor-focused interventions in CBT share much ground with the psychological approach known as coping theory.[11,12] Coping theory is a well-developed and evaluated approach to the stress–response relationship.[13] Elaborating it will assist the case for the materiality of the stressor–depression relationship and how an understanding of that relationship augments autonomy in depression.

6.1.1   Addressing Stressors through CBT: Coping Theory

Coping theory stems from the work of Richard Lazarus and Susan Folkman[14] and is grounded in the tenets of Lazarus' appraisal theory.[15] For a stress response and its related emotions to occur, coping theory holds that a significant goal or interest of the agent must be at stake:

If there is no goal commitment, there is nothing of adaptational importance at stake in an encounter to arouse a stress reaction. Without a stake in one's well-being in any given transaction, stress and its emotions will not occur.[16]

Stressors, on this account, are subject to primary and secondary appraisal. In primary appraisal the individual classifies a stressful interaction as comprising harm, loss, threat, or challenge.[17] Lazarus defines "harm/loss" as "damage that has already occurred" and "threat" as "the possibility of such damage in future."[18] "Challenge" is a more positive response where the testing encounter is framed as an opportunity for the individual to prove himself or herself.[19] The nature of the primary appraisal determines the emotional content of the initial response to the stimulus. Consider the primary appraisals of two students confronted with an unexpected assignment. The student who has done poorly in that subject appraises the new stimulus as "threat" and responds with anxiety. The student who enjoys, and has excelled in the subject deems the additional workload a "challenge" and responds with excitement and curiosity.

In secondary appraisal, the individual examines his or her options for coping with the "stressful person–environment relationship."[20] Lazarus and Folkman define coping as "[c]onstantly changing cognitive and behavioral efforts to manage specific external and/or internal demands that are appraised as taxing or exceeding the resources of the person."[21] The authors propose two types of coping strategies, problem-focused and emotion-focused coping. Problem-focused coping is characterized in the following way:

[A] person obtains information about what to do and mobilizes actions for the purpose of changing the reality of the troubled person–environment relationship. The coping actions may be directed at either the self or the environment.[22]

In the case of the students facing an extra assignment, a problem-focused approach might include seeking an extension to its due date or obtaining information about where relevant resource material could be found. Emotion-focused coping differs in that, rather than manipulating the stressor, it aims to directly target and modify the distressing emotional response:

The emotion-focused function is aimed at regulating the emotions tied to the stress situation—for example, by avoiding thinking about the threat or reappraising it—without changing the realities of the stressful situation.[23]

In the student example, emotion-focused coping might involve distractions such as music or relaxation through exercise or meditation. Ultimately, an effective combination of problem- and emotion-focused coping modifies the stimulus interpretation inherent in the primary appraisal. Thus, the student who initially appraised the extra assignment as threatening might, after seeking guidance from the teacher, now approach it as a challenge. As a consequence, anxiety can be reduced and greater confidence instilled.

Several further elements are integral to coping theory. First, Lazarus emphasizes its transactional nature. Thus, stress results not from a single disposition inherent in either a stressor or its percipient but from a dynamic relationship between the two.[24] Second, stress occurs when situational demands outweigh the individual's coping resources. Lazarus illustrates this point using a "seesaw" analogy, where unchecked demands tip the seesaw to a stressful imbalance when coping is inadequate.[25] Third, stress arises in circumstances that involve the individual's important interests and commitments. The varying nature of personal goal hierarchies means that stressors are often idiosyncratic. Finally, the theory sees stress as emblematic of a person–environment relationship that, unless effective coping occurs, is ultimately maladaptive. At this point, depression is invoked as a signpost indicating that the individual has failed to adapt in the face of a stressful life event.[26] This last point requires elaboration. The Lazarus account sees stress, and related affective states like depression, as outcomes of an agent's inadequate response to contingencies that threaten his or her important interests:

Regardless of how they are defined or conceptualised, the prime importance of appraisal and coping processes is that they affect adaptational outcomes. The three basic kinds of outcomes are functioning in work and social living, morale or life satisfaction, and somatic health. Simply put, the quality of life and what we usually mean by mental and physical health are tied up with the ways people evaluate and cope with the stresses of living.[27]

Thus, on this account "adaptational outcomes" refers to stressor responses that advance the individual's interests in several areas. A point that is emphasized by this aspect of coping theory, and one that I will return to in the next section, is that depression, as a maladaptive stressor response, generally sets back the individual's interests across a number of domains.

A further important element in coping theory, and in CBT, is problem solving. Problem solving is central to problem-focused coping and is a means of altering the stressful person–environment relationship. The overarching goal of problem solving is to revisualize the stressor as a problem with a solution instead of seeing it as an insurmountable obstacle. Donald Meichenbaum has outlined the specific elements of the problem-solving approach:

1. Define the stressor or stress reactions as a problem-to-be-solved.
2. Set realistic goals as concretely as possible by stating the problem in behavioral terms and by delineating steps necessary to reach each goal.
3. Generate a wide range of possible alternative courses of action.
4. Imagine and consider how others might respond if asked to deal with a similar stress problem.
5. Evaluate the pros and cons of each proposed solution and rank order the solutions from least to most practical and desirable.
6. Rehearse strategies and behaviors by means of imagery, behavior rehearsal, and graduated practice.
7. Try out the most acceptable and feasible solution.
8. Expect some failures, but reward self for having tried.
9. Reconsider the original problem in light of the attempt at problem solving.[28]

In depression, situational stressors may respond to problem-focused intervention. Consider the following example. Javier is a busy executive who, faced with increasing work demands, begins spending longer periods away from home. Time spent with his wife and young children is eroded. Gradually, tension builds at home and at work as he increasingly fails to meet expectations in both areas. Sensations of stress give way to depression. Javier seeks help from a psychotherapist with expertise in CBT and problem solving. Together, they determine that a primary source of stress is Javier's immediate superior, who has assigned him an increasing number of exacting tasks. There have also been thinly veiled references to Javier's "expendability" should the demands not be met. The therapist encourages Javier to no longer view the situation as intractable but instead as open to resolution. Javier's priorities are clarified, and it is agreed that, while the job is important, it is untenable in its current form. An assertive approach to the employer is learned and rehearsed, and contingency plans are formulated in the event that Javier should be dismissed. In fact, Javier is retained and his employer begins to show him greater deference, aware now that excessive demands will not be tolerated. Over time, Javier's depressive symptoms ease and his personal relationships improve.

It is important to acknowledge limitations in the application of coping theory to depression. Of most concern is the paucity of data that explicitly link this theoretical model to improved outcomes in depression.[29] However, in a sign the knowledge gap is being addressed, a recent study of over 24,000 Japanese adults from the general population found the use of problem-focused coping strategies to be associated with reduced rates of depression.[30] Moreover, there is now considerable evidence that problem-solving therapy is effective in depression, and it is well established that Lazarus's model forms an important conceptual underpinning of this approach.[31] It is reasonable, therefore, to see coping theory as a valid template with which to conceptualize the specific elements of cognitive therapy that address stressors. Elaborating this approach provides a foundation for the argument to come—that understanding implicit in problem-focused coping is material to the autonomy with which depressed people address stressful life events.

6.2   How CBT Promotes Autonomy in Depression—Addressing Stressors

I now want to argue that CBT, incorporating the kind of stressor-focused approach taken in the example of Javier, promotes autonomy in depression. The argument centers on two claims. The first claim, alluded to and expanded on in chapter 4, is that stressful triggers are likely to relate to the depressed person's principal interests. The second claim is that depression represents a maladaptive, or dysfunctional, response to those stressors. It follows, I will argue, that the depressed person's response to stressors has a potential to impact negatively on his or her important interests. Given that related facts—stressors as depressive triggers, the agent's maladaptive response to them, and the possible remediation of that response through therapy—all pertain to the individual's interests, I will further argue that they are likely to be material to that individual. I conclude that being apprised of those material facts, through therapy, augments the autonomy of the depressed person's associated decisions and actions.

In the previous section, Lazarus measured the adaptational outcomes of problem-focused therapy in terms of well-being, social function, and physical health. I suggested these parameters could also be characterized in terms of the agent's interests, in that most people attach value to successful outcomes in each domain. Effective problem-focused coping can, therefore, be construed as protection, or satisfaction, of the agent's important interests across one or more of these categories. For example, Javier is likely to have a strong, and perhaps urgent, interest in relieving the distressing affective symptoms of depression such as lowered mood, reduced energy, and loss of pleasure. He is also likely to have an interest in the return of adequate functioning in the workplace and at home. A problem-oriented therapy that addresses workplace stress will, in all likelihood, improve not just mood but also job performance, bringing financial security with its attendant benefits. A similar approach to interpersonal issues at home, in addition to improving Javier's affective symptoms, assists the recovery of a healthy spousal relationship, which, in turn, is a boon to his children. In order to see how this aspect of CBT is instrumental in promoting autonomy, it is useful to look again at the concept of materiality.

In chapter 2, I showed that material facts are those with the potential to impact on the agent's important interests. I introduced Gideon, who was confronted with the choice of coronary bypass surgery or medication for heart disease.[32] His principal interests included a writing career, playing tennis, and jogging. Aspects of surgery or medication that might frustrate or advance those interests were shown to comprise material facts. The treating physician was, therefore, guided by Gideon's deeply held values in deciding what facts ought to be conveyed to him during the informed consent process. These observations are also applicable to the individual with depression who attends a doctor. Should the physician wish to ascertain facts that are material to that person, about depression and its treatment, establishing the nature of his or her principal interests will be instructive. The physician should then determine what aspects of depression, and its treatment, are likely to impact on those interests. I have argued that negative affective responses tend to arise when interests are threatened, and triggers of depressive episodes have been alluded to as posing such a threat. It follows that the physician wishing to elucidate facts that are material to the depressed person could make significant progress by investigating triggers for the depressive episode. This reasoning is a summation of the more detailed case for the materiality of the stressor–depression relationship made in chapter 4.

For Javier, workplace and personal stressors have elicited strong negative affect, signaling those domains as integral to his interests. Of course, this is hardly surprising as most people give high priority to these areas. What is significant is that *specific* aspects of those domains have figured in the development of depression and that depression itself indicates Javier's *response* to be maladaptive and counter to his associated interests. It is the potential setback to interests that emphasizes the materiality of the stressor–depression relationship. It is likely to be material to Javier, for example, that his interpersonal dealings with his superior are now so awry that they have contributed to depression. This stressor not only represents a risk factor for serious illness but also indicates a facet of Javier's life requiring special attention to avert related adverse consequences. It follows that information about interventions to deal with stressors, such as problem-focused therapy, would also be material to him.

There is additional reason to hold that depression as a maladaptive response to stressors, and the potential of problem-solving approaches to assist, would be material to the depressed person. Two facets of depression itself, rumination and negative attributional style, can directly impair problem-solving ability. Rumination is prominent in depressive symptomatology. According to Nolen-Hoeksema, it consists in "repetitively focusing on the fact that one is depressed; on one's symptoms of depression; and on the causes, meanings and consequences of depressive symptoms."[33] Evolutionary theory proposes that rumination is a sequel to intense but unsuccessful cognitive efforts to overcome a major threat or difficulty.[34] Others explain it as prompted when vulnerable people face a discrepancy between an existing and a desired state of affairs. Thus,

[w]hen goals cannot be met, and especially if the goal is afforded high value, then the mind will continue to dwell on the discrepancy and search for possible ways to reduce it, giving rise to rumination.[35]

Good evidence suggests that rumination presents a major obstacle to effective problem solving in depression and may, in fact, prolong depression through this effect.[36,37,38] It has been suggested that rumination can be terminated only if the goal in question is attained or if the individual abandons its pursuit.[39] However, mindfulness, an aspect of CBT discussed in chapter 4, seems to afford an additional means of reducing rumination. It brings about a disengagement from the intrusive negative cognitions that feature in this dysfunctional thought pattern.[40]

Negative attributional style also counters the depressed person's ability to effectively address stressors. As explained in chapter 4,[41] this characteristic of depressive thinking leads individuals to assign primary responsibility for negative outcomes to themselves rather than to any inherently taxing properties of a triggering stressor. This trait is antithetic to effective problem solving, in that environmental factors are not ascribed significant causal importance by the depressed individual and, hence, are not seen as suitable targets for problem-based intervention.

Rumination and negative attributional style render the individual susceptible to the depressogenic effects of psychosocial stressors. They are also impediments to effective problem solving in relation to those stressors. It is evident, then, that such response styles have a strong potential to set back the depressed person's interests. CBT addresses rumination through mindfulness techniques. It also addresses negative attributions through "collaborative empiricism," described in chapter 5 in reference to the bank manager whose negative self-attributions were challenged, and ultimately given up, through a consideration of alternative explanations.[42] Their close relevance to interests means that an understanding of these thought patterns, and how they might be remediated, is usually significant for the depressed person.

To summarize, depression, as an affective response, delineates facts about stressors as material to the depressed person. Of most importance are the fact that stressors precipitate depression, the fact that rumination and negative attributional style mediate a maladaptive response, and the fact that problem-oriented strategies can mitigate their effects. The materiality of these facts is emphasized by the multitude of interests that hinge on how well they are understood. These interests relate to the stressful precipitant and the effectiveness with which it is resolved and also to the unfolding depression and the success with which its progression is interrupted. CBT instills understanding of these material facts, enabling a more autonomous stressor response, which, in turn, works to preserve interests and permit the agent greater control over ensuing events. It is my contention that the nature and extent of the autonomy gains seen with CBT are superior to those seen with ADM alone in depression. To advance this claim, it is necessary to offer an account of how treatment with ADM addresses the psychosocial stressors that trigger depression.

6.3   Mode of Action of ADM in Depression—Addressing Stressors

ADM seems to confer resilience to the depressogenic effects of stressors.[43] Precisely how this action occurs is uncertain. However, enough is known about the neurobiological effects of ADM to posit some plausible mechanisms.

6.3.1 The Neurobiology of ADM Action in Depression

In chapter 4, I referred to the hippocampus, a structure located in the brain's limbic system, where emotions are processed.[44] I described how the hippocampus is known to atrophy in the presence of cortisol, a hormone whose levels increase in response to stress. Further, hippocampal atrophy is present in a significant percentage of those with depression. These findings have led some scientists to take the view that stress triggers depression through cortisol-mediated hippocampal atrophy.[45]

ADM has been shown to cause hippocampal neurogenesis, that is, new growth of neurons, in rats.[46] Animal studies have also shown that ADM can prevent stress-induced loss of hippocampal neurons.[47] In addition, it is known that the hippocampus has wide connections to other brain structures that are implicated in symptoms of depression, and it has been proposed that the therapeutic effect of ADM is mediated through those connections.[48] For example, the hippocampus has links with the amygdala, a limbic structure that is active when fear and anxiety are expressed. As outlined in chapter 5, heightened amygdala activity occurs in depression and may mediate some of the effects of negative information-processing biases, for example, tendencies to interpret comments or facial expressions as unpleasant or aversive.[49] In addition, the amygdala's connections with cortical brain structures have been proposed as pathways for the expression of ruminative and guilt-oriented thought patterns.[50] Also, recent data have linked the hippocampus with the brain's reward and pleasure center, the mesolimbic region.[51] It is plausible that effects in this area are responsible for the anhedonia, or loss of pleasure, that prevails in depression. The effects of ADM on the hippocampus and amygdala, and an understanding of their connections with other brain structures, make it reasonable to conclude these to be primary sites of ADM action. Thus, through direct targeting of the limbic region, ADM might dampen a range of depressogenic stressor responses that comprise the individual's diathesis for depressive disorder. These include negative and self-referential information-processing biases, rumination, and the lethargy which can derail the activity scheduling central to behavioral intervention. The relevant neurobiology provides a footing from which to understand the tolerance to stressors afforded by ADM. However, analysis of the autonomy that ADM may confer on the depressive's stressor response is assisted by a fuller account, one informed by clinical experience. The work of psychiatrist Peter Kramer provides a useful illustration in this regard. To picture the effects of ADM within Kramer's framework, it is necessary to look more closely at his view of depression and the role that stress plays in it.

6.3.2   Peter Kramer's Account of Depression

In *Against Depression*, Kramer argues that depression is, in many cases, an organic disease underpinned by a failure of "neuroresilience" in the face of stressors.[52] His view stems from associations between depression and several medical conditions. For example, strokes affecting the frontal area of the brain, especially the orbitofrontal cortex, can trigger "vascular" depression.[53] In addition, interferon treatment for hepatitis C can result in depressive symptoms.[54] And Cushing's syndrome, characterized by an overproduction of cortisol, is also strongly linked to depression.[55] Kramer alludes to the work of Kenneth Kendler,[56] invoking early life trauma as setting the scene for vulnerability to depression in later life.[57] He cites research, described here in chapter 4,[58] suggesting that abnormalities in the serotonin transporter gene are a risk factor for depression.[59] On Kramer's view, and consistent with a diathesis–stress model, depression is often stressor related but manifests in vulnerable individuals:

Depression has a firm biological basis. It is grounded in the genes and in early environmental influences that stand distinct from the psychological. It is progressive, with recurrence leading to heightened vulnerability. . . . At the same time, depression arises from experience. Stressful life events, such as child abuse, lay a groundwork for the sorts of deprivation and failure that lead to illness. Humiliating losses trigger episodes. For many sorts of harm, predisposition matters.[60]

For Kramer, depression represents a "stuck switch" where stress becomes chronic and is associated with unchecked cortisol secretion that damages the hippocampus. Ultimately there is reduced resilience in the face of life's adversities.

The stuck-switch model of depression imagines that a system designed to protect the body [the stress response], acutely, turns on chronically and begins to attack cells and organs it was meant to shield. In this regard, depression is like the autoimmune diseases, such as lupus.[61]

The "neuroresilience" that Kramer contends is conferred by ADM bolsters the individual's coping resources, making the individual more sanguine in the face of loss or other undesirable outcomes. ADM reduces a sensitivity to stress that has both innate and acquired origins. Kramer notes that neuroprotective actions on the hippocampus may mediate the ability of ADM to "mute" stressor responses.[62] His view has common ground with a "permissive theory" of depression.[63] On this account, lowered serotonin does not cause depression directly but permits injuries that do. There is a helpful analogy in his book:

Maybe serotonin is the police. The police aren't in one place—they're not in the police station. They are a presence everywhere. They are cruising the city—they are right here. Their potential presence makes you feel secure. It allows you to do many things that also make you feel secure. If you don't have enough police, all sorts of things can happen. You may have riots. The absence of police does not cause riots. But if you do have a riot, and you don't have police, there is nothing to stop the riot from spreading.[64]

Kramer's account offers a hypothetical but plausible model of ADM action that helps to conceptualize its effects. In light of these and the preceding data, ADM seems to confer resilience to the depressogenic effects of psychosocial stressors. It probably does so by modulating neurotransmitters, which, in turn, alter hippocampal communication with the amygdala, the mesolimbic system, and the orbitofrontal cortex. As a result, the constellation of mood-based, cognitive, and behavioral symptoms that constitute depression are ameliorated. A sound understanding of the mechanism of ADM action provides a grounding to examine its effects on autonomy and to make a comparison with those of psychotherapy.

6.4   Comparing the Effect of CBT and ADM on Autonomy in Depression—Addressing Stressors

In section 6.2 I argued that CBT promotes the autonomy of the depressed person's decisions concerning triggering stressors. I emphasized that stressor-oriented facets of CBT include its problem-solving approach and its capacity to reduce both rumination and negative self-attributions. In order to compare the effects of CBT and ADM on autonomy in depression, some understanding of the cognitive effects of ADM is required. In particular, does ADM augment problem-solving ability, or does it reduce rumination and negative attributional style in depression? Unfortunately, limited data exist with which to address these questions. One review concluded that ADM had negative, neutral, or positive effects on a range of cognitive indices that did not specifically include rumination or attributional style.[65] A further study found a small effect to impair memory and psychomotor performance with various ADMs but concluded that effect to be clinically insignificant.[66] Some work suggests that CBT might be superior to ADM in reducing rumination.[67] However, while authors of a recent review suggest that "antidepressant medication . . . likely reduce[s] ruminative thoughts directly," they concede that more research is needed.[68]

Given the paucity of data, I will, for the sake of argument, grant that ADM *could* reduce rumination and negative attributions and improve problem-solving ability. It seems reasonable to do so in light of the account of ADM action presented in the preceding section and in conjunction with the findings of Catherine Harmer's group on the debiasing effects of ADM, detailed in chapter 5.[69] For example, debiasing through ADM could plausibly act on negative self-referential cognitions in depression. If so, a reduction in negative attributional style might follow. Also, ADM acts on the hippocampus, which, as mentioned in section 6.3.1, has connections with both amygdala and cortex. It has been proposed that the amygdala, through its action on cortical areas involved in memory, might be responsible for rumination.[70] These findings give some neurobiological support to the notion that ADM could improve rumination. Finally, in light of the effect of rumination to retard problem-solving ability, it seems reasonable that if treatment with ADM limits rumination, it might also enhance problem solving in depression. If ADM does exert these effects, a prima facie case exists for its potential to augment the autonomy of the depressed person's stressor-related decisions and actions. To see this, it is important to recall the role played by justified epistemic appraisals in autonomous decision making. Autonomy is construed here as self-determination, encompassing domains of agency and liberty. The agent acts on desires and values that are truly his or her own, a process facilitated by freedom from obstacles and the provision of necessary resources, encapsulated, respectively, in the notions of negative and positive liberty. However, agency and liberty rely crucially on a sound epistemology to ensure that actions cohere with the individual's broader values and more specific desires. Material understanding is necessary if the agent is to choose means that are indeed likely to realize his or her preferred ends. It seems apparent that if ADM reduces negative self-attributions, more justified appraisals of stressors could follow. If rumination is reduced, and problem solving enhanced, there will be more realistic evaluations of the difficulties that must be overcome if the agent's goals are to be met. ADM could, therefore, enhance the prospects that justified epistemic appraisals are made, furthering autonomy with its attendant benefits. As explained previously, those benefits include preservation of interests and greater effective control in the setting of adversity. In sum, it seems possible that ADM could promote the autonomy of the depressed person's stressor-related decisions and do so to an extent comparable to that seen with CBT.

However, there is reason to be cautious in embracing this proposition. It must be remembered that, despite its other effects, treatment with ADM alone does not further the depressed person's *understanding* of the stressor–depression relationship. This difference is pivotal to a comparison of the respective effects on autonomy of ADM and CBT in depression. I have already shown, in section 6.2, how an understanding of the role of stressors in depression augments the autonomy of the depressed person's associated decisions. I held that it is likely to be material to the depressed person that stressors have precipitated his or her illness. The information is material not only because it pertains to a risk factor for serious illness but also because the illness itself sets back the individual's interests in relation to the stressor. I further argued that understanding this information marks stressors as warranting special attention in order to protect the interests at stake and that problem-solving elements of CBT can mediate such outcomes. Accepting this argument, the depressed person treated with ADM alone, who is not apprised of the stressor–depression relationship, takes decisions in relation to triggering stressors that are less autonomous than if the relationship were clear to him or her. Because this assertion derives from an empirical claim about what is *actually understood*, it is not challenged by the fact that the ADM-treated person might demonstrate, incidentally, a greater capacity for problem solving. It is material understanding *that* stressors cause depression, *how* information-processing biases skew stressor appraisals, and *what* problem-focused approaches can achieve in mitigating their effects. Material understanding is the epistemic grounding for autonomous action, that is, action that is most likely to deliver outcomes that cohere with agential values, preserve interests, and evince control. This understanding prefixes the agent's decisions on stressors in a way that plausibly shifts his or her response strategy. For example, knowledge that a particular incident is implicated in depression causation might *motivate* the agent to problem solve in relation to it. By contrast, incidentally improved problem-solving ability via ADM, in the absence of informed motivation, may remain a dormant capacity. By analogy, consider the asthmatic smoker who is meticulously trained in the numerous strategies for giving up cigarettes. Imagine, too, this person is denied the knowledge that smoking exacerbates asthma and remains ignorant of this fact. While this person's capacity to give up smoking is greatly enhanced by the education program, the autonomy with which the person embarks on that course, or resiles from it, is seriously undermined by a poor understanding of the effect of smoking on asthma. The augmented ability to quit is largely redundant in the absence of material information, which is required if the individual's values, goals, and interests are ultimately to be served and furthered by the course of action chosen. Similarly, for Javier, the executive considered earlier, knowledge of the link between stressors and depression will materially inform decisions, for example, to seek alternative employment, to confront his employer, to use relaxation techniques, and so on. Because that understanding is integral to CBT, and could only be obtain felicitously in the person treated solely with ADM, it is CBT that promotes the most autonomous stressor-focused decisions.

Nonetheless, it might still be objected that such understanding is possible, in a depressed person treated with ADM alone, by informing this individual of the broad connection between stressors and depression. For example, the physician might provide a brochure that reads as follows:

You are suffering from depression. You might be especially vulnerable to depression, but it is also possible that a stressful life event has triggered it; most likely it is a combination of the two factors. Cognitive behavior therapy (CBT) can show you how stress contributes to depression. It can also help you better deal with stressful life events. Through therapy, you can learn to recognize how sad feelings cause unrealistic pessimism and how to manage those feelings. CBT is as effective as medication for the type of depression you have.

Prima facie, it seems that the brochure, by informing the depressed person about the stressor–depression relationship, as well as the treatment option of CBT, augments the autonomy of that individual's decisions concerning stressors. If so, then treatment with ADM, and provision of a pamphlet like this one, might augment autonomy to the degree that I contend is seen with CBT.

However, there are problems for such a claim. In particular, there are difficulties with the broad nature of the information contained in the brochure. Consider the case of a person contemplating surgery who is given a similar pamphlet detailing aspects of the proposed operation. To approximate the CBT pamphlet, a representative sentence in the surgical leaflet might read "Surgery has potential side effects that, should they occur, could impact on important areas of your life" or "Surgery can benefit your quality of life and prevent deterioration of your current condition." It is clear that such statements do not contain enough detail to allow the patient to make an autonomous choice about surgery. The patient is likely to be interested in the *precise* risks and benefits of surgery and the *specific* areas of his or her life that would be affected should a particular outcome occur. The more value the individual accords a faculty that is potentially affected by surgery, the more likely it is that he or she will deem the relevant risk or benefit to be material. Overly general information makes it difficult for patients to discern facts that are material to them.

In chapter 2, I alluded to Faden and Beauchamp, who argued for the importance of dialogue in determining aspects of a procedure that are material to the person contemplating it.[71] Conversation, they held, is an effective instrument for unearthing a patient's important goals and values. To achieve adequate "informational exchange," the physician must

ask questions, elicit the concerns and interests of the patient or subject, and establish a climate that encourages the patient or subject to ask questions. This is the most promising course to ensure that the patient or subject will receive information that is personally material—that is, the kind of description that will permit the subject or patient, on the basis of his or her personal values, desires, and beliefs to act with substantial autonomy.[72]

Consider someone who visits a doctor after a finger injury. An X-ray shows the finger to be broken with a slight angulation of the two fragments. Most fractures of this nature can be treated with a simple splint, and there is no need to correct the angulation. However, the person in this case is a concert pianist, and the angulation, although minor, could impair her playing. As a result, for this patient, surgery carries great potential benefit. Ultimately, she decides the risk–benefit calculus favors surgery. For the concert pianist, the exchange of *specific* information with her physician has allowed a determination of what is material to her and an autonomous choice about surgery.

In a similar way, CBT promotes autonomy through the understanding of a *specific* stressor and the individual's maladaptive response to it. That process occurs within the framework of the depressed person's unique life circumstance. Broad information, such as that provided in the brochure about CBT, does not elicit the particular stressors that are implicated in depressive episodes, nor does it delineate the idiosyncratic interests that might be threatened as a result. Moreover, consistent with Faden and Beauchamp's approach, the therapeutic setting in which CBT is delivered facilitates the kind of dialogue necessary to discern the depressed person's peculiar values and concerns. It thus helps elucidate aspects of pertinent life circumstances that may be causal candidates in the depressive episode and amenable to problem-focused remediation. To illustrate, imagine executive Javier is provided with the leaflet on CBT described above. In virtue of what mechanism is he likely to deduce that employer pressure is a preeminent stressor? How is he to determine whether negative self-attributions are active in his interpretation of that stressor? If negative biases are active, will the pamphlet assist him in debiasing a view that his own inadequacies prevent him from meeting the boss's expectations? In the absence of specifically identified stressors, will he be motivated to use problem solving in areas that might be causally related to his depression? It is implausible that such particular details will come to light from a simple reading of the pamphlet information. On all these counts, a more credible thesis is that CBT offers the superior route to material understanding.

In sum, the autonomy promotion seen with CBT is not matched by that achieved through treatment with ADM, alone or in combination with generic information about the stressor–depression relationship. However, there remain further objections to the claim that understanding depressogenic stressors through CBT promotes autonomy to a greater extent than does treatment with ADM. I turn to these now.

6.5   Understanding of the Relationship between Stressors and Depression Promotes Autonomy: Objections

6.5.1   The "Nonshared Environment" Objection

Studies of identical twins frequently aim to determine whether a given trait results more from a genetic or from an environmental influence. In this kind of study, it is important to isolate an environmental factor to which only one twin is exposed. Because identical twins share 100 percent of their genes, if exposure correlates with an increased incidence of the trait under investigation, then reason is adduced for environmental rather than genetic causation. These kinds of factors are said to contribute to the twins' *nonshared* environment, which, as John Rushton explains, includes

all those variables that are unique to each child (e.g. an accident, illness, or chance friendship that happens to one sibling and not to the other); they make people growing up in the same family different from one another.[73]

Conversely, *shared* environment encompasses

all those variables that children reared in the same family have in common (e.g. father's occupation, family cultural practice, parents' child-rearing style); they make people growing up in the same family similar to one another.[74]

However, the notion of nonshared environment is more complicated than this distinction makes out. Nonshared environment also includes effects of shared circumstances that are experienced in unique ways. For example, identical twins might be affected quite differently by parental divorce even if, to an outside observer, it seems they have had equivalent exposure to it. Peter Kramer explains it this way:

The measure for whether an environment is shared, for a given outcome, is whether identical twins respond to it identically—that is, whether they are concordant for the outcome. In many cases, discordant outcomes point to obvious differences in what the twins encounter.[75]

Nonshared environment, then, can be inferred by the presence of "discordant outcomes" when there is no discernible difference in the relevant environment to which an identical twin pair has been exposed. Kramer goes on to explain how this might occur:

For a host of reasons, from intrauterine incidents to the vagaries of fortune on the playground, by age five, even with a shared pair of 5-HTTs[76] and every other gene, one identical co-twin may be confident and the other insecure. Then, a given level of parental support will be adequate for the first and insufficient for the second. In both the experiential and the statistical sense, the home environment is non-shared. That category applies even if the parents swear up and down that they have treated their children identically.[77]

As Kramer notes, Kenneth Kendler's studies showed that the early environmental influences that predict later depression are largely nonshared in this latter sense.[78] Thus, "When background factors, like the tenor of family life, play a role, they do so via the manner in which they are experienced."[79] Kramer uses these findings to argue that when stress causes depression, that interaction depends more on the individual's vulnerability than on taxing properties of the stressor. He puts it this way:

For depression, the environment that matters is the sort that affects different people differently. It is probably true that unattuned parents, indifferent schoolteachers, and poverty cause depression—but only in certain people. When depression is the outcome under study, the effect of overarching, seemingly uniform environments is always, always mediated by the perceiving mind and the predisposed brain.[80]

On my reading of it, Kramer's view constitutes an important objection to the claim that understanding the stressor–depression relationship augments autonomy in depression. While Kramer's account recognizes the role played by stressors, it places great emphasis on diathesis, or individual vulnerability, as a precipitating factor in depression. On this "disease" model, two individuals might be exposed to an identical stressor, yet depression will manifest in the one with, as Kramer phrases it, "underlying physiological defects (like a deficit in resiliency factors or a small hippocampus)."[81] Depression is likened to eczema, asthma, and multiple sclerosis, which are exacerbated by stress but manifest only in those with predisposition.[82] As I see it, this construal holds stressors to be material only in light of their ability to precipitate disease. I have acknowledged this to be a reason to accord material status to an understanding of stressors in depression. However, I have also emphasized that, despite its classification as a disorder, there is a utility in depression that lies in its residual appraisal function, a property it shares with other emotions. Depression is a signal that its trigger threatens agential interests on a host of levels, not just as harbingers of disease. On my reading, Kramer underplays this appraisal facet, reducing depression to an unproductive disorder that might simply be staved off by keeping stressors at bay. In so doing, he presents a counter to the view that stressors, as objects of an emotional response, warrant close consideration because they jeopardize interests. This weakens the case for the materiality of stressors, instead suggesting that strong negative affect, rather than warning of threat or loss, is merely an unfortunate interpretation of a life event, appearing courtesy of aberrant physiology. If stressors are concerning only as etiological agents in disease, rather than as dangerous to interests on a range of other levels, their materiality seems diminished. It is consistent with this view that problem-focused attention to stressors is less important and that efforts to correct flawed physiology are paramount. If the materiality of stressors is lessened, the autonomy gains I hold to flow from their understanding are called into question.

However, there are reasons to think that the autonomy argument I have proposed might resist the objection inherent in Kramer's formulation. To see this, I want to use an example, by analogy, of one of the more common anxiety disorders, social phobia. Individuals with social phobia have an excessive fear of what other people might think of them. This can lead to withdrawal from social situations, impaired function at work, depression, and substance abuse. Although most people have proportionate concern about how others perceive them, the person with social phobia sees negative judgment and criticism where there is none. As a result, it is difficult to see the stressor of social exposure as having a concrete negative impact on the social phobic's important interests. Of course, consistent with the preceding discussion, social exposure does comprise a threat to the agent's interest in avoiding anxiety. However, this narrow threat seems very different from the wide interests at stake when anxiety is provoked by, for example, a partner's threat of divorce, an employer's ultimatum to increase work output, a failing financial investment, borderline grades in a university course, an injury that could bring down an athletic career, and so on. In each of these cases, a range of interests, apart from the desire to avoid distressing feelings, is tied up in how the individual tackles the critical circumstance. Moreover, each trigger seems amenable to problem-focused strategies that might protect broader interests as well as lessen anxiety. Thus, relationship counseling, assertiveness training, financial assistance, individual tutoring, or a second medical opinion might all contribute to stressor resolution. Conversely, because the stress of social exposure seems so distinct from the agent's broader interests, problem-focused interventions, directed at manipulating the stressor, seem not to carry the same potential to preserve threatened interests. It is conceded that established phobia interventions such as graded exposure to fearful events might be construed as a problem-focused strategy. However, the aim here is purely to lessen anxiety rather than to defend a raft of other, equally weighty concerns. On my reading, Kramer's account of depression shares the characteristics of social phobia described here. Depressed people have a heightened sensitivity to minor adversity, whose threat to their significant interests is, at best, difficult to discern. If I interpret him correctly, Kramer would not accord the materiality to stressors in depression that I hold is their due.

One response to this objection is that depression simply is not as Kramer construes it, and not like social phobia. The emotions associated with depression, rather, validly index environmental events as antithetical to interests, whereas the anxiety of social phobia has little utility in this regard. I think I have made a fair case for the claim that depression, despite its maladaptive elements, functions to delineate life events that warrant the agent's scrutiny and thus designates their associated facts to be material. However, I want to take a different tack in addressing this objection and defend the materiality of stressors even granting Kramer's view. If the salience of stressors is shown to be plausible on an account that places heavy emphasis on diathesis, the case for their materiality, and that they merit special attention, is strengthened. To this end, I want to suggest that, even in the case of the social phobic, it is possible to see a legitimate stressor operating. It is widely held that what the phobic is most afraid of is not the apparently fearful situation but his or her own emotional response to it.[83] It is conceivable that the social phobic fears his or her own anxious response, including somatic symptoms such as sweating and palpitations, as much, or more, than the negative judgments of others. Those with phobias often view these symptoms as uncontrollable and possibly the prelude to fainting or a heart attack. There is also the fear of embarrassment and humiliation, should symptoms be evident to others at work or in different social situations. These concerns have a far more plausible basis as threats to the individual's significant interests than the mere presence of other people. It is understandable that, in the setting of anxiety, sweating, and palpitations, an individual might believe there to be a serious underlying medical issue. It is also easy to see that someone whose peers value confidence and self-control would have a strong interest in maintaining an unflustered demeanor. That interest is legitimately threatened by unpleasant feelings and sensations and the potential loss of composure that might follow. Thus, it might be that social situations trigger a cascade of anxieties with a more realistic basis than those inherent in the social circumstance itself. Those concerns can be countered through interventions that focus on the stressor, which, in this case, comprises the individual's own thoughts and feelings. For example, in those who fear that sweating and palpitations herald a heart attack, various strategies can be employed that are directed at challenging the fearful thoughts and lessening the uncomfortable symptoms.

Even if depression is cast as a disease of diathesis, it is, I contend, similarly plausible to identify material stressors as active. Consider the situation, alluded to earlier, of identical twins facing parental divorce, one of whom becomes depressed while the other carries on relatively unscathed. It is quite possible that the vulnerable twin manifests depression after recasting the stressor in a more threatening light. Perhaps the experiences of peers, or the popular media, lead her to extrapolate a more distressing trajectory from her parents' separation. She might envisage loneliness, enduring distress, an impoverished relationship with her parents, and worsening school performance, influenced by knowledge of the plight of a friend or the subject of a magazine article. The salient point here is that the twin's concerns about her parent's divorce relate to plausible potential harms. Each of the hypothesized outcomes can be reasonably expected to occur in some cases. Thus, even in the setting of heightened vulnerability, triggering stressors can reflect realistic threats to interests. Moreover, they might be amenable to targeted interventions focusing, for example, on their actual, rather than feared, probability.

Strong negative affect tends to result from threats to the agent's interests. If the agent perceives threat, or loss, where another perceives none, a reasonable explanation is that he or she has conceptualized the triggering event differently. That subjective interpretation does not diminish the significance of the stressor to the individual. At the very least, stressors that are reframed as overly taxing might truly qualify for that assignation through a self-fulfilling prophecy. The twin who experiences parental separation might indeed suffer the loneliness and distress that she dreads—in virtue of an ensuing affective disorder. A problem-focused, psychotherapeutic approach can, therefore, protect agents' substantive interests by exploring the basis for their perception of a stressor. The action of depressive triggers thus maintains its materiality to the depressed person, despite variations in individual sensitivity. Understanding this, through psychotherapy, can augment the autonomy of the depressed person's related decisions.

6.5.2 A Neuroanatomical Objection

A further possible objection to the contention that understanding the stressor–depression relationship promotes autonomy in depression relates to the neuroanatomical correlates of each treatment for depression. Recall that damage to the hippocampus, probably mediated by stress and the cortisol response, can be repaired by ADM. Neuronal growth in the hippocampus co-occurs with resolution of depression. If ADM restores neurons in areas of the brain associated with psychological resilience, does this imply some advantage in its therapeutic effect? For example, is the action of ADM more enduring? If so, then it might be argued that ADM has a greater autonomy-promoting effect than has been allowed thus far.

However, it is likely that psychotherapy can exert a similar effect on the hippocampus in depression. Admittedly, the evidence for this is circumstantial, as it is much harder to simulate the effects of psychotherapy than to administer a drug in an experimental animal model. However, the empirical findings supporting this claim are persuasive. It is known that nonpharmacological factors can result in hippocampal neurogenesis in laboratory animals. Exercise, environmental enrichment, and electroconvulsive therapy, known to have beneficial effects in animal models of depression, all increase growth of hippocampal neurons.[84,85] Investigations have shown that mice subject to running on a wheel for 4–10 days had significant increases in neuronal growth in the dentate gyrus of the hippocampus.[86] Exercise, especially running, also helps depression in humans.[87] A recent study found chronically stressed rats evinced hippocampal atrophy and "behavioral depression," or immobility.[88] Both hippocampal and behavioral changes were reversed with environmental enrichment, comprising interconnected pipes permitting exploratory behavior and social interaction. Further, as has been alluded to, stress triggers cortisol-mediated hippocampal atrophy and concomitant depression.[89] Psychotherapy, in particular CBSM, acts to improve depression[90] with an associated reduction in cortisol levels.[91] The conclusion that hippocampal atrophy might also be reversed, to some degree, seems reasonable. Finally, some evidence suggests that CBT is more effective in preventing depressive relapse than ADM.[92] If this finding is robust, then ADM action on the hippocampus does not appear to confer advantage in terms of duration of effect. Overall, animal studies showing ADM-induced hippocampal neurogenesis do not present a significant challenge to the autonomy argument favoring CBT.

In summary, psychosocial stressors that trigger depression have a significant potential to impact negatively on the interests of the depressed person. Depression is a dysfunctional response that amplifies the threat posed by stressors. I have argued that, as a result, facts concerning the stressor–depression relationship are likely to be material to the depressed person and that the depressed person who understands those facts is afforded greater autonomy in his or her stressor-related decisions. I showed that CBT engenders such understanding, whereas treatment with ADM alone does not. I concluded that the autonomy of decisions made in depression, in relation to stressors, is promoted to a greater extent through treatment with CBT than through treatment with ADM alone. I suggest, in addition, that the kind of understanding I argue is achieved through CBT involves the depressed person adopting a certain attitude to his or her negative affect. Rather than viewing depressed affect as confirmation of one's own irremediable failings, CBT encourages the individual to view it as an indication of stressors that are legitimately taxing and that can be effectively addressed. The autonomy effects seen with CBT, then, are mediated, at least in part, by the depressed person's holding justified beliefs about the evidential value of his or her affective response.

However, even accepting that CBT is more effective at promoting autonomy in depression, it remains to be shown that an obligation exists for the medical practitioner to prescribe it. It is well established that respect for patient autonomy underpins the informed consent process, which pertains to how a patient *chooses* a particular treatment. However, it is not clear that autonomy promotion ought to be the goal, or the guiding principle, *of the treatment itself*. Thus, although an obligation exists for doctors to respect and promote patient autonomy through adequately informed consent, it is not obvious that doctors are similarly obliged, when deciding between treatments of the same efficacy, to recommend the one that better promotes patient autonomy. This is an important concern, and my response to it forms the basis for the next chapter.

7 A Special Duty to Promote Autonomy in Depression: The Moral Case for Psychotherapy

I'm now going to argue that physicians have a moral obligation to provide CBT to their depressed patients, based on its superior capacity to promote autonomy in this disorder. To make my case, two primary claims must be substantiated. First, it is necessary to show that autonomy promotion is a legitimate and indeed a principal goal of treatment in this disorder. Otherwise, patient autonomy might simply be seen as a factor in the physician's decisions, albeit an important one, without qualifying as a major determinant of treatment choice. In support of this claim, I invoke "parity of reasoning" to show that autonomy promotion in depression is consistent with existing, normatively defensible medical practice. Drawing on clinical examples of antenatal counseling and chronic disease self-management, I show that autonomy promotion is now routine in medicine and is, by parity, also warranted in depression. However, even with this claim established, it remains to be shown that physicians have a duty to promote patient autonomy in depression to the degree seen with CBT. While acknowledging that ADM can further autonomy in depression, I have argued that CBT promotes autonomy to a greater extent and in a different way. Yet, given that ADM does promote autonomy to some degree, it is necessary to demonstrate that doctors have a duty to do more than this. This second claim is substantiated by appeal to the principle of proportionality. I draw on data describing the high relapse rates in depression to argue that autonomy promotion through CBT is quantitatively commensurate with the autonomy threat this disorder poses for sufferers. Finally, I address the objection that a number of competing principles might displace autonomy as guides to management in depression. I discuss the tension between an imperative to promote autonomy and respect for the autonomous wishes of patients who reject CBT in favor of ADM. I also allude to the possibility that beneficence may mandate ceding to an autonomous patient preference to pursue pharmacotherapy in depression.

However, I show the importance of autonomy promotion in depression is sustained in spite of these objections, before concluding that doctors are under a moral imperative to recommend, and enable access to, evidence-based psychotherapy for their depressed patients.

7.1 Parity of Reasoning Supports Autonomy Promotion as a Goal of Treatment in Depression

I want now to use "parity of reasoning" to justify autonomy promotion, through psychotherapy, as a legitimate goal of treatment in depression. Parity of reasoning holds that if the structure of an argument is such that its conclusions are justified, and the structure of a second argument is sufficiently similar in all relevant respects, the conclusions of the second argument are also justified.[1] This principle is also known as "consistency" and relates closely to the adage "Treat like cases alike." The moral force of parity of reasoning stems from the concern that ethical judgments become meaningless if they are inconsistent across cases. For example, it makes little sense to hold someone culpable for driving at excessive speed and then to exonerate another on the basis of his or her superior steering ability. If no morally relevant difference exists between cases, an ethical judgment that holds for one applies also to the other. Prowess at the wheel of an automobile falls short as a moral discriminator, and thus the "better driver" is also subject to speeding laws. I want to show now that autonomy promotion is a normatively defensible treatment goal in a number of medical settings. I want further to show that provision of CBT in depression is sufficiently similar to these examples in relevant moral respects. I will then invoke parity of reasoning to conclude a normative case exists to promote autonomy in depression through psychotherapy.

7.1.1 Parity Argument I: Psychotherapy to Promote Autonomous Consent to Medical Treatment

In recent times, counseling has been used to promote patient autonomy in relation to the informed consent process. Counseling is increasingly recommended for those contemplating termination of pregnancy, particularly in cases where late termination is requested. It is also used to assist those considering reproductive options in the setting of a prenatal diagnosis of genetic abnormality. In the United Kingdom, the Royal College of Obstetricians and Gynaecologists affirms counseling as a priority in both domains:

In the case of late termination in particular, appropriate counselling and safe care for women during this emotional time remain essential. Quality information and counselling are also important prior to antenatal screening and related interventions, in order to prepare women and families for abnormal results.[2]

In addition, genetic counseling is now a benchmark prior to predictive testing for disorders like Huntington's disease. Also, for people considering gender reassignment surgery, psychotherapy is recommended for varying periods, depending on regional codes of practice:

Psychotherapy can provide support for coping with external stressors, treat comorbid conditions, provide increased insight into personal history and motivations, facilitate exploration of the options for living with one's gender identity and enhance decision-making regarding gender transition options.[3]

A primary goal of counseling is to identify the values of the individuals concerned. In this way, material aspects of the test or treatment can be discerned, discussed, and understood, facilitating autonomous decision making. Consider an expectant couple faced with a prenatal diagnosis of Down syndrome. Counseling would explore issues surrounding the disorder including the scope of physical and intellectual disability, associated medical conditions and their treatment, the experience of families raising children with Down syndrome, and the nature and psychological sequelae of termination of pregnancy.[4] The materiality of this information will be a function of how it impacts on the couple's values. They will attach personal significance to, for example, a child's ability to reach independent function, the effects of a disabled child on siblings, the strain such a child may place on the spousal relationship, the child's potential impact on the career of a parent, and so on. Understanding these issues will form the epistemic grounding for accord between the agent's actions and his or her values, goals, plans, and interests. In the setting of rational capacity and requisite freedom, the provision of this material information will enhance the autonomy of a decision to continue with or to terminate the pregnancy.

I want to show now that parity of reasoning can be applied to these examples in a way that grounds a normative case for the use of CBT in depression. To do so, two claims must be substantiated. First, it must be shown that the promotion of autonomous choice through genetic and antenatal counseling is normatively defensible. Merely showing such counseling to be a common or even benchmark clinical practice does not, on its own, show it to be ethically required. Second, the action of CBT in depression to promote autonomy must be demonstrated to be sufficiently similar to these examples in relevant moral respects. If the two cases are not substantially alike, parity cannot be invoked to confer moral equivalence.

The first claim is established by reference to arguments for the value and normative force of autonomy. Recall that autonomy holds value on two counts. On the instrumental view, autonomy derives value from the capacity of autonomous choice to further the agent's good or well-being. On this account, well-being equates with the satisfaction of rational and informed preferences. Autonomous individuals, in virtue of their critical and reflective capacities, freedom from impediments to action, and possession of appropriate resources, are well placed to achieve this notion of the good. The intrinsic value of autonomy, on the other hand, notes the importance of exercising control over events, even when that course is less likely than another to increase well-being. The normative force of autonomy can be explained in terms of each category of value. On the instrumental account, autonomy promotion is ethically compelling because of the emphasis we place on personal well-being. Our concern for the individual's good is moral motivation to expedite his or her autonomous choices. In the medical realm, concern for the good of patients is formalized in the physician's duty of beneficence. The connection between autonomy and the good forms the basis for a moral imperative that physicians, bound to act in their patients' best interests, work to promote patient autonomy. On the intrinsic view, it is respect for persons that drives the normative force of autonomy promotion. Because persons are agents with broad and intensely held interests that can be both thwarted and furthered, persons are vulnerable to being wronged. This trait leads to the association of personhood with moral status and, consequently, the view that the choices of those who qualify as persons warrant respect. Because the capacity for autonomy is elemental to personhood, respect for persons extends also to respect for their autonomous choices.

Thus, the normative force in promoting autonomy through genetic and antenatal counseling derives from a concern for both patient well-being and empowerment. On the instrumental account, autonomous choices about proceeding with or terminating a pregnancy in the setting of Down syndrome are likely to result in outcomes that accord most closely with patient interests. Autonomy promotion is, therefore, consistent with, and perhaps a requirement of, the physician's duty to act in the patient's best interests. On the intrinsic view, respect for autonomous choice is mandated by a concomitant imperative to respect persons. If autonomous choice requires dialogue to elicit material information, then respect for persons implies a duty to hold this conversation. Autonomy promotion is a necessary step if the couple in question is to make an autonomous health care choice. On the intrinsic account, the exercise of autonomous choice retains value independent of the well-being attached to its outcome.

There is a formidable moral case to promote patient autonomy through the provision of counseling in the instances detailed. However, to complete the argument from parity of reasoning, it remains to be shown that CBT in depression is similar in critical moral respects. A pivotal semblance between psychotherapy in depression and genetic counseling is that both promote autonomy by eliciting material facts. Material information is that with the potential to have an impact on the agent's dominant interests. This point has been made at length, and I will not belabor it here. However, I do want to emphasize a related observation. The elucidation of material information indicates the target life circumstance to hold crucial significance for the individual. Understanding aspects of raising a child with Down syndrome, or undergoing a pregnancy termination, is material because it pertains to life-altering choices. Similarly, many decisions in depression relate to triggering stressors which are delineated, by the depressive response itself, as significant life events. CBT imparts information that is material because it contributes to how stressors are addressed and because it is crucially relevant to the success of that process. Autonomy promotion in both genetic counseling and psychotherapy for depression occurs in relation to life events whose potential consequences are onerous, cementing the moral parallels between them.

A second salient commonality is that doctors who treat depression, as with those offering genetic testing, antenatal screening, and related medical treatments such as pregnancy termination, owe their patients a duty of care. Under this duty, doctors must strive to act in their patients' best interests. Autonomy promotion subserves this goal in that autonomous patients are uniquely situated to advance their interests. It might reasonably be concluded that autonomy promotion through counseling, and hence through CBT for depression, is required by the normatively uncontentious duty of care that applies universally to doctors. However, some may object that such a conclusion ignores a relevant distinction. The counseling example establishes a normative case to promote autonomous *consent* to treatment, whereas CBT promotes autonomy through the *treatment* of depression itself. On this objection, parity is not made out because the similarity criterion is breached in a way that is, arguably, morally relevant. Thus, the objection holds, a duty to promote autonomous consent does not, without further argument, also support a duty to promote more extensive autonomy through medical treatment.

In reply, I propose that a doctor's duty of care indeed extends to the depressed patient's life decisions, distinct from the informed consent process. Further, it follows that autonomy promotion in relation to broader life matters is consistent with, or required by, the doctor's duty of care. To see this, consider one of the diagnostic elements of major depression, the presence of suicidal thoughts or plans.[5] Unsurprisingly, their diminution or disappearance is, all else equal, an indication of effective treatment. Doctors are therefore bound, under their duty of care, to reduce suicidal thinking in depressed patients. Patently, a decision to take or to desist from taking one's own life is frequently made outside the medical realm in the domestic environment. A doctor's duty of care plausibly extends, therefore, to intensely personal decisions that are distinct from the consent process. It is not difficult to come by other examples. Specialists in drug and alcohol rehabilitation influence patients to limit substance use, nutrition consultants entreat obese patients to eat healthily and to exercise, hypertension experts exhort patients to reduce salt intake, and so on. In such cases, if no attempt were made to influence the patient's life choices, there would be a dereliction of the doctor's duty of care. To extend this duty to the promotion of patient autonomy, recall its value as an instrument to patient well-being. On the basis of this connection, doctors aiming to advance patient interests are bound to promote the autonomy of wider, health-related, life choices. Because this goal is inherent in the psychotherapeutic treatment of depression, duty of care can be legitimately brought to bear as the basis for a moral imperative to promote patient autonomy in this disorder. In consequence, there is little merit in the objection that a doctor's duty to promote autonomy applies only to consent and not to treatment.

In sum, counseling to promote autonomous consent to treatment is an existing, ethically justified medical practice. The promotion of autonomy through provision of CBT in depression bears similarity in critical ethical respects. There is, therefore, a persuasive argument from parity of reasoning for a moral imperative to provide psychotherapy in depression.

7.1.2 Parity Argument II: Autonomy Promotion through Medical Treatment Itself

To consolidate the argument that doctors face a moral imperative to promote autonomy through treatment, and not just in relation to informed consent, it is possible to invoke a second parity of reasoning example. I want to show now that doctors already institute *medical treatments* that aim largely at autonomy promotion. I will also show such treatments to be normatively defensible, that CBT in depression possesses descriptive similarity, and, therefore, that parity of reasoning supports an ethical case to provide it.

Consider the increasingly prevalent condition of diabetes mellitus. Type I diabetes generally appears in childhood or adolescence and requires life-long compliance with a regime of insulin injections to ensure adequate blood sugar control. As a result, it is also known as insulin-requiring diabetes. Type II diabetes typically occurs later in life and is associated with overweight and obesity. It is usually managed with diet control, oral glucose-lowering medication, and occasionally with insulin injections, should other measures be ineffective. However, the management of diabetes is not restricted to simple dietary advice or to medication. A significant aspect of care, at least in developed countries, is diabetes education. Most educators are experienced nurses who have completed additional tertiary training. A grounding tenet of this discipline is diabetes self-management education (DSME), which, as its name suggests, aims to enable those with diabetes to manage the illness with minimal dependence on health care providers.[6] DSME has a number of components. Through it, patients learn about the influence of various food types on blood sugar, as well as more general nutritional principles. They are informed about the effect of exercise to reduce blood sugar and how weight loss can diminish the requirement for medication or insulin. DSME also covers the management of excessively high or low blood sugar. In addition, counseling deals with the psychosocial impact of diabetes. Indeed, through programs based on Stanford University's chronic disease self-management model, this approach is increasingly applied to other conditions, including arthritis and back pain. Bodenheimer and colleagues explain it in the following way:

Sometimes called "patient empowerment," this concept holds that patients accept responsibility to manage their own conditions and are encouraged to solve their own problems with information, but not orders, from professionals.[7]

Although DSME aims to improve diabetic control, that goal is clearly associated with an attempt to enhance the autonomous choices of people with diabetes. Rather than simply receiving a drug or an injection that can maintain steady glucose levels, patients are provided with information about diet, exercise, and psychosocial aspects of the illness that allow it to be dealt with in a range of ways. This information relates closely to agential interests and thus qualifies as material. Many facts will, for example, bear on how well diabetes is controlled and, therefore, on the success with which its often crippling complications are held at bay. The knowledge that comes with DSME is also pivotal for those who wish to reduce dependence on medication and minimize their risk of drug side effects. Others may have a particular aversion to self-injection, and thus measures that allow insulin to be replaced with tablets become meaningful. Understanding this material information permits individuals greater autonomy in managing the disorder. DSME demonstrates a medical preference for a treatment with equivalent efficacy to available alternatives, which also strives to enhance patient autonomy.

Again, to show parity between this example and psychotherapy for depression, DSME must be shown to be normatively sound, and the use of CBT in depression must be proven relevantly similar. The normative status of DSME can be ascertained with reference to the earlier discussion on the value of autonomy. Promotion of autonomous choice is driven by a moral imperative stemming from autonomy's instrumental and intrinsic value, respectively, the capacity of autonomous choice to further patient interests and to enhance control. The similarity criterion is satisfied in relation to the parameters of material information, significant life events, and duty of care cited earlier. Both DSME and CBT in depression furnish patients with material facts that inform major life decisions. Moreover, those decisions are acutely relevant to how well a target illness is resolved and thus fall squarely within the remit of the treating doctor's duty of care. Parity of reasoning can, therefore, be invoked to see autonomy promotion through psychotherapy in depression as consistent with an extant and ethically supported medical treatment that also aims to promote autonomy.

I want to preempt the next section by suggesting that a comparison between DSME and depression management also supports my argument for a depression treatment that promotes autonomy to a degree superior to that of its alternatives. Thus, there is little doubt that the autonomy of the person with diabetes benefits from the provision of medication and a glucose-monitoring device alone. The illness can be controlled to a degree that allows the individual, all else being equal, to function at an adequate level. In this respect, such basic measures reflect the degree of autonomy promotion that might be seen in the depressed person treated with ADM alone. However, in diabetes much greater autonomy promotion is achieved through the measures outlined, which are justified by the ethical imperative deriving from the value of personal autonomy. Diabetes management is an example of an existing preference in medicine for a treatment that, among a range of available options, promotes autonomy to the *greatest extent*. Parity also supports, therefore, an ethical obligation to treat depression with the effective option that also promotes autonomy to the greater extent.

The parity of reasoning argument for the use of CBT in depression can be summarized as follows. Psychological counseling, in relation to consent to medical tests or interventions, is already used with the primary aim of promoting autonomy. A strong case suggests this course to be morally defensible. The use of psychotherapy in depression is an effective treatment that also aims to promote personal autonomy. It is relevantly similar to consent counseling because in both instances there is provision of material facts, about significant life circumstances, by physicians who hold a duty of care to the patients in question. Counseling thus supports an argument from consistency, or parity, for a moral imperative to provide psychotherapy in depression. An objection is that CBT for depression promotes autonomy in relation to broad life events rather than specific treatment decisions and is not sufficiently similar to the example of counseling for consent. This claim is rejected on the basis that promotion of autonomous consent is required under a doctor's duty of care, a duty I show extends to patients' wider life decisions and thus to the promotion of autonomous, illness-related choices outside of the consent domain. A second parity of reasoning argument invokes diabetes management as an example of an existing medical treatment that aims squarely to promote patient autonomy. This clinical practice is shown to be morally sound and to set an ethical precedent for autonomy promotion through the use of CBT in depression.

However, while parity of reasoning supports autonomy promotion as a legitimate goal of treatment in depression, more must be said to establish a moral duty for doctors to promote autonomy in depression to the degree seen with CBT. I want to argue now that the magnitude of autonomy lapses in depression makes CBT both a proportionate and a warranted response.

7.2 An Argument from Proportionality for Autonomy Promotion in the Treatment of Depression

It is generally accepted that medical therapy ought to be proportionate to the severity, and the chronicity, of the illness it is intended to treat. This provision can be traced to the doctor's duty of beneficence, which requires doctors to offer treatment that is in the patient's best interests. Part of the calculation preceding medical decisions is a weighting of the relative risks and benefits of an intervention under consideration. The notion of proportionate treatment reflects a balanced appraisal of risks and benefits.[8] Thus, a person with a minor respiratory infection is justifiably advised to rest, use simple analgesia, and perhaps take oral antibiotics. Administration of more intensive treatment, such as intravenous antibiotics, would be disproportionate. While intravenous delivery more reliably achieves therapeutic drug levels, the benefits in such a mild condition are outweighed by its risks, which include infection, blood clots, and drug leakage into surrounding tissue. However, in severe respiratory illness, such as pneumonia, treatment commonly involves hospital admission, intravenous medication and, in critical cases, assisted ventilation. Each of these interventions is associated with considerable morbidity. Even the decision to admit someone to the hospital is risky. A recent meta-analysis found 9.4 percent of hospital patients had an adverse event, usually related to drug administration or a surgical procedure.[9] Nor were these trivial events—7 percent led to permanent disability and 7.4 percent were fatal. However, the high lethality of serious pulmonary infection generally justifies such risks. The notion of proportionate treatment reflects a desire for a successful therapeutic outcome weighed against the incidence and gravity of recognized complications or side effects. Delivery of proportionate treatment is central to the exercise of beneficent care.

How, then, is proportionality to be calculated? There is no simple answer. While there are evidence-based guides to the kinds of treatments known to control given disease states, individuals will place a personal value on percentage rates of success, failure, and adverse outcomes. Appraisals will be influenced by what each person considers material about a given treatment. Consider the nausea and vomiting associated with cancer chemotherapy. In someone for whom treatment is palliative, the impaired quality of life might outweigh the gains of a comparatively small survival extension. On the other hand, for a person with the potential for cure, these unpleasant side effects may seem a small price. While this example shows a significant subjective element to the determination of proportionate treatment, it also suggests an objective or perhaps intersubjective component. Many would judge the risk of side effects from chemotherapy warranted if the prospects were good for an acceptable quality and quantity of added life span.

I want to make a case that the determination of proportional treatment in depression can be deduced though appeal to this kind of analogy. The chronicity of depression, its detrimental encroachment on so many aspects of life, and in particular the magnitude of the threat to personal autonomy it comprises suggest a treatment that promotes autonomy to a greater rather than lesser extent is proportionate. To appreciate the breadth of injury associated with depression, consider some if its characteristics. Those with depression tend to have multiple episodes. On standard definitions, *remission* from depression is regarded as a brief asymptomatic period whereas *recovery* involves a longer period with no symptoms.[10] *Relapse* is defined as the return of symptoms during remission and *recurrence* as the return of symptoms during recovery.[11] It is known that, in those who remain untreated, 50 to 80 percent are likely to have a relapse or recurrence of depression.[12] However, even in those taking long-term antidepressants, the relapse rate is up to 80 percent within five years.[13] Recent data indicate that 76 percent of patients relapse when antidepressants are discontinued after an initial therapeutic response, compared to 47 percent in those who continue to take medication.[14] In the same study, the relapse rate for those who completed CBT as the sole treatment modality was around 31 percent.[15]

The point here is not to show that CBT has a lower relapse rate than treatment with ADM alone, although if this finding can be reproduced, it will certainly have implications for depression treatment on efficacy grounds alone. What these data also show is that depression has a strong potential to run a chronic course. Therefore, all the contingencies that go with depression, from pessimistic biases to psychosocial triggers, are likely to reenter the depressed person's psychological landscape at a later time. The probability of future autonomy threats is high. As a result, the magnitude of potential autonomy gains in depression, through CBT, is substantial. Thus, when a stressor appears, and the person with remitted depression senses a lowering of mood, CBT training ought to make itself felt. That person might respond with a heightened awareness of the role of stressors as an influence on mood and will be more accomplished at using problem-focused methods to address them. Also, a trained skepticism can be brought to bear when predictions veer to pessimism in concert with lowered mood. Understanding these techniques means that decisions made during future depressogenic scenarios will demonstrate greater autonomy than if the person remained untrained in CBT. Of course, the depressed person treated with ADM alone might be more resilient in the face of depressogenic stressors and is perhaps better placed to deal with them. However, without an understanding of the skills just outlined he or she is deprived of an important option for managing potential recurrences. Given that nearly 50 percent of those with depression who are treated with long-term ADM are subject to relapse, the autonomy advantage afforded through CBT becomes even more salient.

The examples cited earlier, of instances where autonomy promotion constitutes a significant goal of patient care, provide substance to a general contention that autonomy promotion can be a legitimate goal of medical treatment. The high incidence of recurrence in depression means that its effects to erode autonomy become an issue of prevention, not just one concerned with an extant episode. As a result, the potential for autonomy impairment, seen as cumulative over a long period of stressor exposure, becomes substantial. This ethical concept has real-life implications for sufferers. Depressed people are plagued by an unhappiness that skews interpretations of relationship difficulties, family issues, and workplace challenges. There is commonly a failure to understand and to identify causal stressors and to use problem-focused strategies to deal with them. The depressed person is unprepared to navigate these situations in a way most likely to see his or her interests well served and to maintain the kind of life control that is a concomitant of well-being. A proportionate treatment is, on the proposed framework, one whose effectiveness is commensurate with the severity of the illness and one that does not impose a risk burden that is excessively onerous. CBT targets the autonomy threat of depression and is thus a treatment that is not only effective on recognized criteria but that works toward patient well-being and empowerment in the longer term. This therapy explicitly addresses the kinds of knowledge and skill gaps that undermine the autonomous response to adverse life events in those with depression. CBT does, therefore, tick a good number of boxes on the benefit side of the proportionality scale. Moreover, the risks associated with it are negligible. While ADM is as effective as CBT and promotes autonomy to some degree, there is a solid case in depression for a treatment that achieves more than this. In addition, ADM has recognized side effects, including rash, diarrhea, nausea, anxiety, and sexual dysfunction, among others. These observations strongly suggest that CBT, or a psychotherapy that embodies its relevant characteristics, comprises a proportionate response to the autonomy threat posed by depression. Further, as detailed earlier, the relationship between autonomy and patient interests means autonomy promotion falls within the scope of the doctor's duty of care. The institution of proportionate treatment is also elemental under a physician's duty of care. On both counts, doctors owe a compelling duty to provide this form of psychotherapy to depressed patients.

Yet, it may still be objected that autonomy is merely one of a number of principles that compete for the doctor's attention as guides to treatment. On this view, autonomy promotion is important but can be displaced by more weighty ethical concerns. If persuasive, this objection could undermine the moral case for CBT in depression, and so it must be addressed.

7.3   An Objection from Competing Principles against Autonomy Promotion as a Treatment Determinant in Depression

In making treatment recommendations to patients, doctors are guided by a number of principles. A reason to accord less importance to autonomy is the presence of a competing principle that carries equal or greater weight in the relevant circumstance. In what follows, I examine some principles that might compete with autonomy as guides to treatment in depression. I conclude that none presents sufficient reason to diminish the importance I ascribe to autonomy promotion as a goal of treatment in depression.

7.3.1   The Proper Goals of Medicine
Could a preference for CBT in depression be challenged by an objection that its property of promoting autonomy is not a proper goal of medicine? If autonomy promotion were considered an inappropriate goal, or perhaps supererogatory to a physician's other duties, the support it gives to an ethical case favoring CBT might be undermined. A closer examination of the goals of medicine is required.

In an influential project of the Hastings Center, led by Daniel Callahan, a multinational task force sought to specify and provide justification for their notion of the proper goals of medicine.[16] They concluded there to be four such goals:

1. The prevention of disease and injury and the promotion and maintenance of health.
2. The relief of pain and suffering caused by maladies.
3. The care and cure of those with a malady, and the care of those who cannot be cured.
4. The avoidance of premature death and the pursuit of a peaceful death.[17]

In defining "health," the group departed from the widely adopted World Health Organization standard of "complete, physical, mental and social well-being,"[18] stating that

[b]y "health" we mean the experience of well-being and integrity of mind and body. It is characterized by an acceptable absence of significant malady, and consequently by a person's ability to pursue his or her vital goals and to function in ordinary social and work contexts. By this definition we aim to stress a traditional focus on

body wholeness and general well-working, on the absence of malfunction, and on the resultant ability or capacity to act in the world.[19]

At first glance the statement of the Hastings Center group seems to be consistent with the goal of promoting patient autonomy. I have defended a view of autonomy that specifies agency, liberty, and epistemic reliability as instruments to the fulfillment of goals that accord with the individual's values. If, as the group specifies, "health" encompasses an ability to pursue vital, individual goals and to act in the world, it would seem to cohere well with the proposed conception of personal autonomy. However, the group seemed at pains, later in the document, to point out that autonomy promotion was not, and ought not to be, a principal goal of medicine:

In one sense medicine has always sought to promote some forms of autonomy, for instance the promotion of a functional autonomy with the physically or mentally disabled. . . . While it is true that health does enhance the possibility of freedom, it is a mistake to think of such freedom as a goal of medicine. Health is a necessary, but not sufficient condition for autonomy, and medicine cannot supply that sufficiency.[20]

I want to make two responses to the claims made here by the task force. First, it is manifestly true that health is necessary but not sufficient for autonomy. We accept that autonomy is a multivariate trait. To be autonomous is, among other things, to possess information, to have the capacity to utilize it, and to be free from unjustified coercion, arbitrary restraint, or ad hoc punishment. It is uncontentious that the satisfaction of these requirements hinges on both a functioning education system and the opportunity to access it. It also requires a robust infrastructure of democratic government subject to appropriate checks and balances. Plainly, medicine, or the broadly construed health that it delivers, is not sufficient for an autonomy that also rests on other foundational pillars. However, it is, as the task force points out, necessary to have a requisite quantum of health to achieve the kind of autonomy that such a society permits. This brings me to my second point. It can be conceded that health is merely a necessary condition for autonomy without ceding autonomy as a proper goal of medicine. It is quite consistent, I maintain, to accept health as necessary for autonomy and also to aim at health for its capacity to confer autonomy. It may be helpful to invoke an example from legal discussions of causation, where scholars sometimes refer to the NESS test, for "necessary element in a sufficient set."[21] If a candidate causal factor satisfies the NESS requirement, it is, accepting the test's validity, duly noted to have caused the outcome under investigation. If *health* satisfies the NESS test for *autonomy*, and autonomy is desired, why can't health be desired because it is instrumental to autonomy, even if it not sufficient to bring it about alone? Accepting this, it is reasonable to hold that autonomy could comprise at least one of the legitimate, and surely very important, goals of health care. Of course, it might still be objected that a goal of promoting autonomy through medicine could be self-defeating in that health, as a mere necessary condition, is required in only a limited quantity for adequate autonomy. However, in the preceding sections I hope to have shown that aiming at autonomy promotion by degrees through various health interventions can make a discernible difference to overall autonomy in everyday life. I also hope to have demonstrated that the value inherent in that difference makes it worth striving for.

A further line of argument also supports autonomy as a proper goal of medicine. Many aspects of what physicians aim at, as a healthy outcome, are closely connected to the individual's personal autonomy. For example, someone facing bilateral below knee amputations after road trauma has two major options to restore mobility; limb prostheses or a wheelchair. The choice will depend on a number of factors including the individual's determination and persistence, innate athleticism, the wheelchair accessibility of local services, desire for upright posture and the appearance of a normal gait, and so on. In this case, the very nature of what a healthy outcome consists in is contingent upon the autonomous choice of the individual. Remember that autonomous choice gives a strong indication of the course of action most likely to further the individual's interests. Thus, the person who, after reflecting on his or her own values and capacities, autonomously chooses to mobilize in a wheelchair, provides the treating doctor with information about what is best for him or her in the circumstance. This input is critical to a decision about the patient's best interests and can only be obtained through an autonomous communication from that patient. Because doctors are duty bound to act in patients' best interests, situations such as this demand a concomitant duty to promote autonomy in order to glean those interests. Autonomy promotion becomes, therefore, a cardinal goal of medicine in virtue of its engagement with beneficent practice.

At this point, an important distinction must be drawn. There may exist a tension between autonomy promotion as a goal of treatment and respect for patient autonomy as a determinant of treatment. Thus, the question arises whether doctors who seek to promote patient autonomy through the provision of psychotherapy should accede to the autonomous requests of depressed patients to receive ADM. If this question is answered in the affirmative, it leads to the somewhat uncomfortable conclusion that respect for autonomy mandates autonomy *not* being promoted in such cases. This is an important concern, as reason suggests autonomous individuals should be the arbiters of the value they attach to the facility of autonomy itself. Admittedly, there are strong utilitarian arguments against agents' undervaluing autonomy through, for example, selling themselves into slavery. On this view, the good that derives from autonomy provides moral reason to ensure that it is not constrained, even as the result of autonomous choice. It is improbable, however, that the same argument could apply to those who resist, through refusal of psychotherapy, promotion of what is already an adequate level of autonomy. Of course, the definition of "adequate autonomy" might eventually alter, perhaps even because of the kind of arguments presented here. However, in the current climate, the depressed person who autonomously chooses ADM over CBT should undoubtedly have that wish respected. Nonetheless, the capacity of CBT to promote autonomy in depression, and how it does so, is information that should be made very prominent in the discussion from which such a choice issues. My argument urges both physician and patient to consider this property of CBT as a morally compelling reason to view it as essential treatment in depression. Thus, while respect for autonomous patient wishes might limit delivery of psychotherapy in individual cases, it does not overturn a normative case for the value of autonomy promotion more generally in those with depression.

There is, in summary, little merit to the claim that autonomy promotion is not a proper goal of medicine. The value of autonomy is such that health becomes a laudable goal in virtue of being instrumental to greater autonomy. Indeed, autonomous choice is a guide to patient's interests, so autonomy promotion can be necessary for an assessment of best interests. This connection confers further legitimacy on autonomy as a goal of health care. While respect for autonomous choice might limit provision of autonomy-promoting therapy in specific cases, the moral worth of personal autonomy as an overarching goal remains. In consequence, CBT cannot be rejected as a morally obligatory treatment in depression, based on a contention that the aim of autonomy promotion lies outside the proper goals of medicine.

7.3.2 Professional Autonomy

Professional autonomy notes the importance of the physician's being free to make decisions based on the knowledge and expertise garnered through professional practice. As Bayles has argued, "If professionals did not exercise their judgment in these aspects, people would have little reason to hire them."[22] As a result, a case might be made that physicians treating patients with depression can rightly appeal to professional autonomy to justify their treatment choice. If this were so, then an appeal to promote patient autonomy in depression, and thus a recommendation to prescribe CBT, might legitimately be resisted by physicians who preferred to prescribe ADM.

Bayles also emphasizes that professional autonomy can be properly limited by the benchmarks or guidelines of the professional's supervising organization.[23] This situation operates in the medical paradigm. For example, an individual practitioner might have a strong and sometimes warranted faith in the efficacy of a treatment that has not been subject to appropriate testing. However, there is a clear expectation that the practitioner will not prescribe it until rigorous studies establish its effectiveness and the relevant bodies approve its use.[24] However, this contingency does not pertain to the case under consideration. Current Australian and international guidelines for the treatment of mild, moderate, and severe uncomplicated depression recommend *either* ADM or psychotherapy, leaving the ultimate choice to the practitioner.[25] Given that the two treatments are accorded equal weight in therapeutic guidelines, it seems reasonable that a practitioner *could* appeal to professional autonomy to justify a treatment choice other than CBT. Many physicians in primary care adopt psychological medicine as a subspecialization. As a result, through short courses, postgraduate diplomas, or seminars, they gain extra knowledge and expertise in the treatment of psychological disorders. That knowledge, combined with a familiarity with their patient's character, can place them in a special position to decide which treatment will be better tolerated, or perhaps more efficacious, in a given individual.

However, there remain reasons to think that exercise of professional autonomy ought to defer to the goal of promoting patient autonomy in these cases. Consider the potential benefits and costs, to doctor and patient, of submitting to professional autonomy, if that favored ADM, or electing to promote patient autonomy through CBT. If professional autonomy were to prevail, the benefits might be measured in a number of ways. There might be physician satisfaction at the ability to determine treatment according to his or her expertise. Further, there is some evidence that the exercise of professional autonomy can be justified on broader, beneficence-based grounds:

[T]he professionals' greater freedom of decision and action becomes the client's and the society's most likely route to the desired results, for in this way uninformed and misinformed lay interference is excluded in favor of the expert's competence. Thus professional autonomy and control of work are presented as being as much a benefit to the client and the society as they are boons to the profession and to professionals.[26]

If this claim were applicable here, there would be good cause to determine treatment according to the physician's choice. To do so would seem to deliver overall net benefit. However, it must be remembered that ADM and CBT are of equal efficacy in common grades of depression.[27] As a result, it is difficult see how an appeal to professional autonomy, in support of treatment with ADM, could be justified on beneficence grounds. Appeals to beneficence could be made to justify *either* treatment.[28] Further, the challenge to professional autonomy presented does not comprise "misinformed lay interference" but rather a carefully elaborated ethical argument. Such a challenge seems unlikely to undermine the physician's exercise of beneficence in relation to his or her depressed patient.

Consider now the cost to the patient if professional autonomy prevails in such a way that ADM is prescribed. The patient is denied the skills with which to make more informed choices in relation to significant life events, potentially impacting on major career and relationship decisions. His or her ability to deal with the future depressogenic effects of stressors is lessened, so that autonomy lapses, and recurrent depression, are more likely to ensue. On the other hand, if promotion of patient autonomy is accorded greatest weight, then, for the reasons just outlined, there is significant advantage to the patient of acquiring the skills that come with CBT. Further, the cost to the physician of promoting patient autonomy does not seem great. She has fulfilled her duty of beneficence and conformed to robust practice guidelines for the treatment of depression. Weighing these considerations, the possibility of limitation to the exercise of professional autonomy does not constitute reason to retreat from autonomy promotion, through CBT, as a goal of depression treatment.

7.3.3 Cost–Benefit Considerations

It is conceivable that an objection might be made to the use of CBT in depression based on an analysis of the relative costs and benefits of available treatments. It might be argued that, although CBT yields an autonomy advantage when compared to pharmacotherapy in depression, CBT should be resisted as the preferred treatment because of its higher initial costs. A typical course of CBT involves one session per week over 16 weeks. In Australia, for example, a full course of CBT with a psychologist in private practice costs around AU $1,840, and with a psychologist in the public health care system, approximately AU $750.[29] In comparison, a standard course of treatment with ADM, lasting 6 to 12 months, costs around AU $250–500.[30] Prima facie, if both treatments are of equal efficacy, then ADM appears to be more cost-effective.

However, this comparison is too simplistic to evaluate the inherent cost–benefit trade-offs. A significant factor ignored is the emerging evidence of reduced relapse rates in those treated with CBT.[31] Thus, while analyses of efficacy data and costs early in the posttreatment phase might support the use of ADM, longer term studies are more likely to favor CBT. Studies that aim at a valid econometric comparison between treatments mostly use the parameter of disability adjusted life years (DALY). A DALY is a measure of the number of healthy years an individual loses to a particular disease and is the unit generally employed to measure burden of disease.[32] A recent Australian study using this parameter concluded that CBT offers favorable cost benefit results compared to pharmacotherapy.[33] For example, treatment with an SSRI antidepressant costs AU $14,000 per DALY saved compared to AU $10,000/DALY for individual CBT with a public or private psychiatrist, AU $8,500/DALY for CBT with a private psychologist, and AU $3,500 for CBT with a public psychologist. The study did find treatment with tricyclic antidepressants (TCA) to be competitively cost-effective at AU $5,500/DALY. However, although TCA remains as a treatment option on standard management guidelines, it is prescribed much less than a decade ago. This probably relates to its significant side-effect profile compared to SSRI and its greater lethality in overdose. Of course, the overall cost of treatment does not always reflect the cost to the patient. However, in Australia access to public psychologists is fully covered by the universal health care scheme Medicare[34] and, since November 1, 2006, 12 visits to a private psychologist are now subject to a rebate. Thus, close to a complete course of CBT is now widely available in Australia.

Examination of cost-effectiveness data from other countries yields varying results. In the United States, Antonuccio and colleagues found that, in treatment of depression, fluoxetine alone resulted in 33 percent greater costs than CBT alone, and a combination of fluoxetine and CBT resulted in 23 percent higher costs than CBT alone.[35] This study did not employ DALY or quality adjusted life year (QALY) methodology. However, Pirraglia and colleagues found a wide variation, based on cost per QALY saved, in the cost–utility of pharmacological (U.S. $3,100–U.S. $34,000) and psychotherapeutic (U.S. $24,000–34,000) interventions for depression.[36] This study was a meta-analysis of nine cost–utility studies in depression and did not look specifically at CBT as the psychotherapeutic modality.

The authors also noted that "most striking is the paucity of cost utility research in depression," highlighting difficulties in gaining accurate data with which to assess relative treatment costs in depression.[37] In the United Kindgom, Layard, citing the evidence from controlled trials showing reduced relapse after CBT, asserts that the cost-effectiveness of CBT and ADM in depression is similar.[38]

While acknowledging that definitive claims await more complete data, it is reasonable to conclude that the cost-effectiveness of CBT is likely to be no worse than, and is probably better than, pharmacotherapy, and so an objection to the provision of CBT on cost–benefit grounds is unpersuasive.

7.3.4   Beneficence

It is a cornerstone of medical practice that physicians strive to act in their patients' best interests. Indeed many hold beneficence to be *the* guiding ethical principle in medicine. Might there be circumstances where, in depression, to promote patient autonomy through CBT would entail the physician failing in his or her duty of care to the patient? That is, could CBT, while promoting autonomy, also *set back* the patient's significant interests? In this case, there would be good reason to assign diminished importance to personal autonomy as a goal of treatment in depression.

Prima facie, such a contention appears to have little substance. In depression, ADM and CBT are of equal efficacy, and, as stated, they are given equivalent weighting in Australian and international guidelines for the management of depression. These recommendations imply that by instituting either treatment the physician fulfills his or her duty of care. However, it is still the case that individual patients could have reason to prefer ADM over CBT. The patient might prefer a treatment that took less time or required minimal alteration to a busy schedule. The patient might place greater weight on relieving the distressing symptoms of depression and less emphasis on addressing potential stressors, or he or she might simply not be "psychologically minded" and have no wish to gain the kinds of insights that come with psychotherapy. In short, the patient might not value the promotion of autonomy that occurs through treatment with CBT.

In such a case, it seems that beneficence could displace autonomy promotion as a guide to the kind of treatment the patient ought to receive. I have argued that the input of a competent patient is important in order to determine treatment that is in his or her interests.[39] I have shown that so-called objective conceptions of the good have little place in guiding medical treatment and, in some cases, can be manipulated to justify strongly paternalistic interventions. Thus, if a patient's fully informed preference were to be treated with ADM, there would be reason, on the account I have presented, to hold such treatment to be in the patient's best interests.

I emphasize, however, that patients must be exposed to information about the merits of psychotherapy. The value and normative force of autonomy is such that doctors are morally required to fully elaborate the nature of CBT before accepting autonomous patient preference as a determinant of best interests. Only after this case has been made, and compared to the risks and benefits associated with ADM, does the patient's decision satisfy the requirements of autonomous consent. I further stress that I do not argue autonomy promotion to trump *all* other concerns in the doctor–patient relationship. What I have aimed to show is that autonomy promotion ought to be a principal goal of treatment, one that is foremost in the concerns of the treating physician faced with a depressed patient. I have argued that autonomy promotion, in the setting of two treatments *of equal efficacy*, provides a compelling moral basis for the prescription of CBT. This argument is premised on the assumption that the physician's duty of beneficence is satisfied through the provision of either treatment. Competent patient preference for ADM sways beneficent practice toward that option, and here the goal of autonomy promotion might be subsumed to the dictates of beneficence. Yet, there remain many cases where beneficence supports either treatment, and so the importance of autonomy promotion should make itself felt, and psychotherapy recommended.

To close, personal autonomy, in virtue of both instrumental and intrinsic value, wields considerable normative force in health care. Autonomy promotion is already a morally defensible goal of the informed consent process and of emerging models of chronic disease self-management. These examples set a precedent for an ethical requirement that doctors promote autonomy through CBT in depression. Further, the magnitude of the autonomy threat posed by depression makes the superior autonomy promotion of CBT, against ADM, a proportionate response. Proportionate treatment is required under a doctor's duty of beneficence, an observation providing further moral warrant for CBT in depression. While ADM prescription may, in some cases, follow from respect for autonomous choice or an assessment of best interests, the broader normative value of autonomy promotion remains. Given that, in most cases, a doctor fulfills his or her duty of beneficence by providing ADM or CBT, the additional capacity of psychotherapy to advance autonomy makes it morally incumbent upon practitioners to provide it for depressed patients. It is now possible to summarize the moral case for psychotherapy in depression and to identify some of the hurdles to its implementation.

7.4   The Moral Case for Psychotherapy and the Way Forward

Doctors who treat depression are undoubtedly dealing with people who have disordered brain chemistry.[40] Prima facie, it might seem that the required treatment ought to be a drug that directly targets neurotransmitters, such as ADM. However, it is crucial to remember that many brain chemicals involved in the regulation of emotion are exquisitely sensitive to environmental change and, in particular, to stressors. Brain chemistry and emotion are context dependent. This observation supports a different approach, one that addresses the context in which the disordered emotion has arisen.

I argue that a critical ethical distinction must be drawn between the pharmacological and psychotherapeutic approaches to depression. That distinction is rooted in the understanding that is gained by the depressed person through therapy and that is largely ignored in purely drug-based management. This knowledge carries decisive ethical weight because, through it, the individual regains personal autonomy, a trait worn perilously thin in depression. It does so by apprising the agent of facts about the contextual nature of depressive disorder. Specifically, therapy furthers understanding that stressors trigger depression, how negative biases mediate their interpretation, and what the agent can do to protect the interests at stake. This knowledge augments the autonomy of major life decisions made by those with depression, outstripping any parallel effect of treatment with ADM alone.

The argument is situated in a wider debate about the nature of emotion. I adduce persuasive philosophical and psychological accounts supporting an evaluative thesis of emotion. Emotions can provide evidence for states of affairs and of the value an individual places on their outcome. However, that evidence can vary in quality. Emotions can reinforce both justified and unjustified beliefs. I characterize this property of emotion as its evidential value. I conclude that the ability to discriminate between emotions with high and low evidential value is vital if the agent is to deal autonomously with the object of the emotional response. I show CBT to confer this ability in depression and, therefore, to more effectively promote autonomy in the disorder. Yet, I concede such a conclusion does not, in itself, entail a duty for doctors to prescribe psychotherapy for depressed patients. However, I argue that depression constitutes a special case and that it requires an autonomy-focused treatment. I support the argument by appealing to the current, justified, ethical weight placed on autonomy in the physician–patient relationship. Most doctors are assiduous in respecting and promoting patient autonomy through, for example, enabling informed consent to medical interventions. I argue that consistency mandates conferring equivalent prominence on autonomy as a goal of treatment in depression. However, the strongest reason for advocating autonomy promotion in depression is the extent to which autonomy is subverted by this illness. Depression is not only a disorder of affect but also a "disorder of autonomy." Rational deliberation and judgments about significant life events are increasingly out of reach as depression worsens. In consequence, a therapy heavily weighted to autonomy promotion is a proportionate, and warranted, response.

Current guidelines for the management of depression in primary care do not recognize the ethical divide that I draw between its two principal treatment modes. Indeed, authors of the Australian guidelines counsel doctors treating depression, "*It is not so much what you do but that you keep doing it.*"[41] In light of the recent, and timely, burgeoning appreciation for patient autonomy in medicine, this is surely a deficiency. Physicians treating patients with mild, moderate, and severe uncomplicated depression have an ethical imperative to prescribe CBT. In consequence, the guidelines as they stand are wanting, in that they fail to reflect the autonomy threat posed by depression and the ability of available remedies to address it.

What is to be done? This book provides a first step by sending a clarion call to practitioners that the provision of self-knowledge in depression is not just a treatment alternative but is a moral matter. Through a psychotherapeutic understanding of the mechanics of depressive illness, sufferers are better able to protect their interests and to prevent control slipping from their grasp. Greater autonomy is not just a slogan but a tangible outcome of considerable value. Doctors who set back the autonomy of depressed people by withholding psychotherapy fail spectacularly in a fundamental ethical obligation. This book will, I hope, sow the ideological seeds necessary to convince practitioners that it is time for a new approach.

Yet there remain obstacles. ADM is squarely embedded in the firmament of depression treatment. A reductionist "biological" mentality prevails that sees deranged neurochemistry as warrant for pharmacological correction, in apparent ignorance of the responsiveness of brain chemicals to environmental manipulation. One can posit a number of driving factors. Direct-to-consumer advertising is a pervasive influence, straight to the lounge room, which poses the question, "Illness?" and invariably inculcates the answer, "Drug." Pharmaceutical companies spend enormous sums disseminating this message, in itself suggesting that advertising is an effective means of increasing medication uptake and profits. A counter strategy could require the equal efficacy of evidence-based psychotherapy to be clearly indicated during drug commercials. For this advice to be effective, however, public awareness of psychotherapy must be raised through media campaigns including television commercials, mailing out of educational brochures, and placement of information leaflets in medical waiting rooms.

Physicians in private practice are also subject to the profit motive. It makes financial sense to deal with a greater number of patients and spend less time with each. Drug prescriptions can now be generated at the press of a button, but delivering psychotherapy, or even explaining it as a treatment option, requires considerable time. This issue might be addressed by rewarding physicians who deliver psychotherapy with remuneration that accurately reflects the required time commitment. Also, primary care training programs could routinely include skills acquisition in cognitive therapy, to widen the pool of clinicians capable of providing it. An additional incentive to provide psychotherapy is the professional satisfaction that often comes with proficiency in a new discipline. However, primary care doctors may simply be too busy to deliver therapy, no matter how well trained or reimbursed. In this setting, a major problem becomes the dearth, in some regions, of specifically trained psychotherapists. This deficiency could be corrected by funding extra positions in university psychology schools for those who pledge to practice in these areas. The mooted scheme is similar to the bonded scholarships that exist in some Australian medical schools, where studies are subsidized on the proviso that graduates will spend a stipulated period working in underresourced, usually rural regions. However, even with the implementation of such measures, if costs to patients remain prohibitive, then uptake of psychotherapy will be hampered. Governments must ensure that psychotherapeutic interventions for depression are subsidized to an extent enabling wide community access. However, if efforts to lobby authorities for funding are to be successful, it is imperative to address the research shortfalls that hamper proper cost–benefit comparisons between psychotherapy and ADM. Solid data confirming CBT to compare favorably to ADM on cost–utility criteria would greatly enhance any case that the state underwrite provision of psychotherapy services.

Perhaps a more intractable hurdle is the widespread desire for a "quick fix." Self-analysis can be painful, protracted, hard. The lure of a pill is that psychic exertion might be avoided, unpleasant introspection made redundant, and a speedy return to business as usual assured. In response, it must be emphasized that cognitive and related psychotherapies are skills oriented, of predetermined duration, and yield validated outcomes. While some exploration of very painful emotional experiences is unavoidable, the emphasis is on modification of "here and now" interpretative processes. Because evidence-based psychotherapy is delivered over a relatively short period, it should be palatable for those concerned about interruptions to busy timetables. It must also be stressed that depression is recurrent, and that if relapse is to be prevented, and indeed if meaning is to be derived from depressive episodes, time must be set aside for those purposes.

Any regulatory response should also aim at young people. Rates of depression are increasing, highlighting the importance of prevention. Emotional intelligence programs are already beginning to operate in schools, teaching children to recognize and manage their own feelings and how best to respond to the emotional states of others. These programs could also cover abnormal psychology and discuss strategies that anticipate and counter the emergence of psychological disorder. Education policy should also target medical schools to ensure that the tenets of evidence-based, nonpharmacological depression treatments are taught alongside drug-oriented strategies. Here, too, the heavy emphasis on pharmacotherapy might be tempered by banning the sponsorship of educational events by pharmaceutical companies. Sales representatives for drug manufacturers are poorly situated to provide balanced information about their products. There is a clear conflict between the interests of objective data presentation and commercial imperatives. The numerous cases of publication bias stemming from suppression of unfavorable trial results attest to this.

Each of these avenues for change is underpinned by the basic ethical imperative asserted in this book. Self-knowledge in depression furthers individual good and empowerment and is, therefore, of pressing moral significance. Autonomy promotion should be a preeminent concern of clinicians working at the front line with depressed patients. The health care professions must recognize the ethical requirement for psychotherapy in depression and embrace the many conversations that are necessary to deliver it.

Appendix: The Hamilton Rating Scale for Depression

Patient Name: _____

Rater Name: _____

Date: _____

Activity   **Score**

Depressed mood   _____

Sad, hopeless, helpless, worthless
0 = Absent
1 = Gloomy attitude, pessimism,
hopelessness
2 = Occasional weeping
3 = Frequent weeping
4 = Patient reports these feelings states in
his/her spontaneous verbal and non-verbal
communication.

Feelings of guilt   _____

0 = Absent
1 = Self-reproach, feels he/she has let people
down
2 = Ideas of guilt or rumination over past
errors or sinful deeds
3 = Present illness is punishment
4 = Hears accusatory or denunciatory voices
and/or experiences threatening visual
hallucinations. Delusions of guilt.

Suicide   _____

0 = Absent
1 = Feels life is not worth living
2 = Wishes he/she were dead, or any
thoughts of possible death to self
3 = Suicide, ideas or half-hearted attempt
4 = Attempts at suicide (any serious attempt
rates 4)

Insomnia, early   _____

0 = No difficulty falling asleep
1 = Complaints of occasional difficulty in
falling asleep—i.e., more than half-hour
2 = Complaints of nightly difficulty falling
asleep

Insomnia, middle   _____

0 = No difficulty
1 = Patient complains of being restless and
disturbed during the night
2 = Waking during the night—any getting
out of bed rates 2 (except voiding)

Insomnia, late   _____

0 = No difficulty
1 = Waking in the early hours of the
morning but goes back to sleep
2 = Unable to fall asleep again if he/she gets
out of bed

Work and activities   _____

0 = No difficulty
1 = Thoughts and feelings of incapacity
related to activities: work or hobbies
2 = Loss of interest in activity—hobbies or
work—either directly reported by patient or
indirectly seen in listlessness, indecision and
vacillation (feels he/she has to push self to
work or activities)

3 = Decrease in actual time spent in
activities or decrease in productivity
4 = Stopped working because of present
illness

Retardation   _____

*Slowness of thought and speech; impaired
ability to concentrate; decreased motor activity*
0 = Normal speech and thought
1 = Slight retardation at interview
2 = Obvious retardation at interview
3 = Interview difficult
4 = Interview impossible

Agitation   _____

0 = None
1 = Fidgetiness
2 = Playing with hands, hair, obvious
restlessness
3 = Moving about; can't sit still
4 = Hand wringing, nail biting, hair pulling,
biting of lips

Anxiety, psychological   _____

*Demonstrated by: subjective tension and
irritability, loss of concentration, worrying about
minor matters, apprehension, fears expressed
without questioning, feelings of panic, feeling
jumpy*
0 = Absent
1 = Mild
2 = Moderate
3 = Severe
4 = Incapacitating

Anxiety, somatic   _____

Physiological concomitants of anxiety such as:
dry mouth, indigestion, diarrhea, cramps,
belching, palpitations, headaches,
hyperventilation, sighing, urinary frequency,
sweating, giddiness, blurred vision, tinnitus
0 = Absent
1 = Mild
2 = Moderate
3 = Severe
4 = Incapacitating

Somatic symptoms: gastrointestinal   _____

0 = None
1 = Loss of appetite but eating without
encouragement
2 = Difficulty eating without urging.

Somatic symptoms: general   _____

0 = None
1 = Heaviness in limbs, back or head;
backaches, headaches, muscle aches, loss of
energy, fatigability
2 = Any clear-cut symptom rates 2

Genital Symptoms   _____

Symptoms such as: loss of libido, menstrual
disturbances
0 = Absent
1 = Mild
2 = Severe

Hypochondriasis   _____

0 = Not present
1 = Self-absorption (bodily)
2 = Preoccupation with health
3 = Strong conviction of some bodily illness
4 = Hypochondriacal delusions

Loss of Weight Rate either 'A' or 'B':

A. When rating by history:
0 = No weight loss
1 = Probable weight loss associated with present illness
2 = Definite (according to patient) weight loss
B. Actual weight changes (weekly):
0 = Less than 0.5 kg weight loss in one week
1 = 0.5 kg–1.0 kg weight loss in week
2 = Greater than 1 kg weight loss in week
3 = Not assessed

Insight

0 = Acknowledges being depressed and ill
1 = Acknowledges illness but attributes cause to bad food, overwork, virus, need for rest, etc.
2 = Denies being ill at all

Diurnal Variation

A. Note whether symptoms are worse in morning or evening.
If no diurnal variation, mark none
0 = No variation
1 = Worse in A.M.
2 = Worse in P.M.
B. When present mark the severity of the variation.
0 = None
1 = Mild
2 = Severe

Depersonalization and derealization

Feelings of unreality, nihilistic ideas
0 = Absent
1 = Mild
2 = Moderate
3 = Severe
4 = Incapacitating

Paranoid symptoms   _____

0 = None
1 = Suspicious
2 = Ideas of reference
3 = Delusions of reference and persecution

Obsessional and compulsive symptoms   _____

0 = Absent
1 = Mild
2 = Severe
TOTAL Score   _____

Source: Hamilton, M. 1967. Development of a rating scale for primary depressive illness. *British Journal of Social and Clinical Psychology* 6 (4):278–96. This version taken from the University of Massachusetts Medical School website at <http://healthnet .umassmed.edu/mhealth/HAMD.pdf>.

Notes

Chapter 1

1. National Center for Health Statistics. 2007. Health, United States, 2007. Hyattsville, MD.

2. Healy, D. 2000. Good science or good business? *The Hastings Center Report* 30 (2):19–22.

3. World Health Organization. 2008. Global burden of disease: 2004 update. Geneva: WHO Press.

4. Ibid.

5. Greenberg, P. E., and H. G. Birnbaum. 2005. The economic burden of depression in the US: societal and patient perspectives. *Expert Opinion on Pharmacotherapy* 6 (3):369–76.

6. Styron, W. 1990. Darkness visible: a memoir of madness. New York: Random House. p. 50.

7. Ellis, P. M., and D. A. Smith. 2002. Treating depression: the beyondblue guidelines for treating depression in primary care. "Not so much what you do but that you keep doing it." *The Medical Journal of Australia* 176 Suppl:S77–83.

8. Australian Institute of Health and Welfare. 2005. Mental Health Services in Australia 2003–2004. Canberra. p. 44.

9. When I refer to antidepressant medication (ADM), I refer to the current, most commonly prescribed categories, namely, selective serotonin reuptake inhibitors (SSRIs) and selective noradrenaline reuptake inhibitors (SNRIs).

10. Australian Institute of Health and Welfare. p. 46.

11. Australian Institute of Health and Welfare. p. 48.

12. National Center for Health Statistics.

13. Stagnitti, M.N. 2008. Antidepressants prescribed by medical doctors in office based and outpatient settings by specialty for the U.S. civilian noninstitutionalized population, 2002 and 2005. Rockville, MD: Agency for Healthcare Research and Quality.

14. National Institute for Health Care Management. 2002. Prescription drug expenditures in 2001. Washington.

15. Ellis and Smith.

16. Hollon, S. D., R. J. DeRubeis, R. C. Shelton, J. D. Amsterdam, R. M. Salomon, J. P. O'Reardon, M. L. Lovett, P. R. Young, K. L. Haman, B. B. Freeman, and R. Gallop. 2005. Prevention of relapse following cognitive therapy vs medications in moderate to severe depression. *Archives of General Psychiatry* 62 (4):417–22.

17. See chapter 4, section 4.5.2, for the derivation of these figures.

18. See the appendix.

19. A formal definition of depression from the *Diagnostic and Statistical Manual of Mental Disorders* is included in chapter 4, section 4.1.

20. Ellis, P. 2004. Australian and New Zealand clinical practice guidelines for the treatment of depression. *Australian and New Zealand Journal of Psychiatry* 38 (6):389–407.

21. While interpersonal therapy is effective in depression and problem-solving therapy demonstrates promising results, I concentrate on CBT because it has been more extensively investigated and its mechanism of action has been more comprehensively elucidated. It is important to state at the outset that the arguments put forward in this book pertain to elements of CBT that might also form part of other therapies. If this were the case, then my arguments would apply, all else being equal, to the other therapies as well.

22. Ellis and Smith.

23. An important qualifier is that a combination of ADM and psychotherapy is likely to be more effective than either treatment alone in the management of chronic depression (symptoms for more than 2 years) of at least moderate severity. See de Maat, S. M., J. Dekker, R. A. Schoevers, and F. de Jonghe. 2007. Relative efficacy of psychotherapy and combined therapy in the treatment of depression: a meta-analysis. *European Psychiatry* 22 (1):1–8.

24. Ellis and Smith.

25. Henceforth, when I use the term "depression," I do so in relation to mild, moderate, and severe uncomplicated major depression, the categories to which my argument pertains.

26. Ellis and Smith.

27. American Psychiatric Association. 2000. Practice guideline for the treatment of patients with major depressive disorder, 2nd ed.

28. American Psychiatric Association. 2005. Guideline watch for the practice guideline for the treatment of patients with major depressive disorder.

29. National Institute for Clinical Excellence. 2007. Depression (amended): management of depression in primary and secondary care. London: NICE (Clinical Guideline 23).

30. Around two-thirds of depressive episodes are triggered by identifiable psychosocial stressors, a point I expand on at length in chapters 4 and 6. See Kendler, K. S., L. M. Karkowski, and C. A. Prescott. 1999. Causal relationship between stressful life events and the onset of major depression. *American Journal of Psychiatry* 156 (6):837–41.

31. Ibid.

32. Some writers, most notably Randolph Nesse, have argued that depression may have adaptive utility in facilitating disengagement from futile goals, procuring care from close friends and family, and inhibiting the hasty take-up of new plans at times when the individual is poorly placed to realize them. While not discounting Nesse's claims, my argument draws on the considerable morbidity and mortality associated with depression to frame it as, in many cases, a formidable threat to the agent's interests. See Nesse, R. M. 2000. Is depression an adaptation? *Archives of General Psychiatry* 57 (1):14–20.

Chapter 2

1. Dworkin, G. 1988. *The theory and practice of autonomy, Cambridge studies in philosophy*. Cambridge; New York: Cambridge University Press. p. 12.

2. Beauchamp, T. L., and J. F. Childress. 1994. *Principles of biomedical ethics*. 4th ed. New York: Oxford University Press. p. 121.

3. Berlin, I. 1969. Two concepts of liberty. In *Four essays on liberty*. Oxford: Oxford University Press.

4. Young, R. 1986. *Personal autonomy: beyond negative and positive liberty, Croom Helm international series in social and political thought*. London: Croom Helm. p. 7.

5. Dworkin, p. 14.

6. Beauchamp and Childress, p. 121.

7. Dworkin.

8. Frankfurt, H. 1971. Freedom of the will and the concept of a person. *Journal of Philosophy* 68 (January):5–20.

9. For a discussion of hierarchical models of autonomy (also termed "coherence" models), see Buss, S., Personal autonomy. In *The Stanford encyclopedia of philosophy (Fall 2008 edition)*, edited by E. N. Zalta. <http://plato.stanford.edu/entries/personal-autonomy>.

10. Taylor, J. S. 2005. Introduction. In *Personal autonomy: new essays on personal autonomy and its role in contemporary moral philosophy*, edited by J. S. Taylor. Cambridge: Cambridge University Press.

11. Watson, G. 1975. Free agency. *The Journal of Philosophy* 72 (8):205–20.

12. Christman, J. 1991. Autonomy and personal history. *Canadian Journal of Philosophy* 21 (1):1–24.

13. Mele, A. 1993. History and personal autonomy. *Canadian Journal of Philosophy* 23 (2):271–80.

14. Young, *Personal autonomy: beyond negative and positive liberty*, p. 8.

15. Fischer, J. M., and M. Ravizza. 1998. *Responsibility and control: a theory of moral responsibility, Cambridge studies in philosophy and law*. Cambridge; New York: Cambridge University Press.

16. Christman, J. 2001. Liberalism, autonomy and self-transformation. *Social Theory and Practice* 27 (2):185–206.

17. Berofsky, B. 1995. *Liberation from self: a theory of personal autonomy*. Cambridge; New York: Cambridge University Press. p. 135.

18. Swinburne, R. 2001. *Epistemic justification*. Oxford: Oxford University Press. p. 72.

19. Ibid., p. 138.

20. Faden R. R., T. L. Beauchamp, and N. M. P. King. 1986. *A history and theory of informed consent*. New York: Oxford University Press. p. 254.

21. Benson, J. 1983. Who is the autonomous man? *Philosophy* 58:5–17.

22. Ibid.

23. Ibid.

24. Young, *Personal autonomy: beyond negative and positive liberty*, p. 12.

25. Ibid., p. 12.

26. Buss.

27. Taggart, D. 2002. About impaired minds and closed hearts. *British Medical Journal* 325 (7375):1255–6.

28. Faden, Beauchamp, and King.

29. Ibid., p. 303.

30. Skene, L., and R. Smallwood. 2002. Informed consent: lessons from Australia. *British Medical Journal* 324 (7328):39–41.

31. Rogers v Whitaker. 1992. 67 ALJR 47.

32. Faden, Beauchamp, and King, p. 302.

33. Ibid., p. 307.

34. This point will be considered in more detail in section 2.4.

35. Theories of the value of autonomy are discussed in detail in section 2.4.

36. Pellegrino, E. D., and D. C. Thomasma. 1988. *For the patient's good: the restoration of beneficence in health care.* New York: Oxford University Press. p. 7.

37. Ibid., p. 5.

38. Ibid., p. 13.

39. Neil, D. A., S. Clarke, and J. G. Oakley. 2004. Public reporting of individual surgeon performance information: United Kingdom developments and Australian issues. *The Medical Journal of Australia* 181 (5):266–8.

40. Ibid.

41. Buchanan, A. E. 1978. Medical paternalism. *Philosophy and Public Affairs* 7 (4):370–90.

42. Ibid.

43. Ibid.

44. Buchanan, A. E., and D.W. Brock. 1990. *Deciding for others: the ethics of surrogate decision making.* Cambridge: Cambridge University Press. pp. 29–30.

45. Buchanan.

46. "Competence" is a legal term that equates to the possession of "decision-making capacity." Briefly, a competent patient is one who can comprehend, believe, and reason in light of information material to a proposed medical intervention, before choosing whether to consent to it. Accounts of competence tend to align with epistemic construals of autonomy but generally eschew consideration of desire-based theories. A competent medical decision can thus be considered, roughly, the legal analog of an autonomous medical decision. See Stewart C., and P. Biegler. 2004. A primer on the law of competence to refuse medical treatment. *Australian Law Journal* 78:325–42.

47. Griffin, J. 1986. *Well-being: its meaning, measurement, and moral importance.* Oxford: Clarendon Press. p. 8.

48. Parfit, D. 1984. *Reasons and persons*. Oxford: Clarendon Press. p. 493.

49. Griffin, p. 8.

50. Ibid., p. 11.

51. Ibid., p. 40.

52. Buchanan and Brock, p. 36.

53. The authors are referring here to mental state, desire-based, and objective theories of the good.

54. Buchanan and Brock, p. 35.

55. Feinberg, J. 1971. Legal paternalism. *Canadian Journal of Philosophy* 1 (1):105–24.

56. Woodward, J. 1982. Paternalism and justification. *Canadian Journal of Philosophy; Supplementary volume* 8:67.

57. Feinberg.

58. Woodward.

59. Styrud, J., S. Eriksson, I. Nilsson, G. Ahlberg, S. Haapaniemi, G. Neovius, et al. 2006. Appendectomy versus antibiotic treatment in acute appendicitis: a prospective multicenter randomized controlled trial. *World Journal of Surgery* 30 (6):1033–7.

60. Mill, J. S. 1974. *On liberty*. New York: Meridian. p. 138.

61. Ross, L., and R. E. Nisbett. 1991. *The person and the situation: perspectives of social psychology*. Philadelphia: Temple University Press. p. 238.

62. World Medical Association. 2009. *Declaration of Helsinki: ethical principles for medical research involving human subjects* 1964 [cited August 30, 2010]. <http://www.wma.net/en/30publications/10policies/b3/index.html>.

63. Beecher, H. K. 1966. Ethics and clinical research. *New England Journal of Medicine* 274 (24):1354–60.

64. Young, R. 1982. The value of autonomy. *The Philosophical Quarterly* 32 (126):35–44.

65. Ibid. Quote from: Brandt, R. B. 1959. *Ethical theory: the problems of normative and critical ethics*. Englewood Cliffs, NJ: Prentice-Hall. p. 303.

66. Glover, J. 1977. *Causing death and saving lives*. Harmondsworth; New York: Penguin. p. 81.

67. Wiggins, J. S. 1996. *The five factor model of personality: theoretical perspectives*. New York: Guilford Press. p. 98.

68. Allen, N. B., and P. B. Badcock. 2003. The social risk hypothesis of depressed mood: evolutionary, psychosocial, and neurobiological perspectives. *Psychological Bulletin* 129 (6):887–913.

69. Young, R. *Personal autonomy: beyond negative and positive liberty.* p. 31.

70. Ibid., p. 31.

71. Pettit, P. 1993. Consequentialism. In *A companion to ethics*, edited by P. Singer. Oxford: Blackwell.

72. Alexander, L. Deontological ethics. In *The Stanford encyclopedia of philosophy (Fall 2008 edition)*, edited by E. N. Zalta. <http://plato.stanford.edu/entries/ethics-deontological>.

73. Kant, I. 1965. *Fundamental principles of the metaphysic of ethics.* Translated by T. K. Abbot. London: Longmans. p. 55.

74. Ibid., p. 56.

75. Tooley, M. 1972. Abortion and infanticide. *Philosophy and Public Affairs* 2 (1):37–65.

76. Ibid.

77. Gruen, L. The moral status of animals. In *The Stanford encyclopedia of philosophy (Spring 2009 edition)*, edited by E. N. Zalta. <http://plato.stanford.edu/entries/moral-animal>.

Chapter 3

1. For a survey of theories of emotion, see the opening chapter of Prinz, J. 2004. *Gut reactions: a perceptual theory of emotion.* New York: Oxford University Press.

2. See, for example, Nussbaum, M. 2003. Emotions as judgments of value and importance. In *What is an emotion?*, edited by R. Solomon. New York: Oxford University Press; Solomon, R. C. 2004. Emotions, thoughts, and feelings: emotions as engagements with the world. In *Thinking about feeling: contemporary philosophers on emotions*, edited by R. Solomon. New York: Oxford University Press; Goldie, P. 2004. Emotion, feeling, and knowledge of the world. In *Thinking about feeling: contemporary philosophers on emotions*, edited by R. Solomon. New York: Oxford University Press.

3. Kelly, T. Evidence, *The Stanford encyclopedia of philosophy (Fall 2008 edition)*, edited by E. N. Zalta. <http://plato.stanford.edu/archives/fall2008/entries/evidence>.

4. Gardner, T. J., and T. M. Anderson. 2009. *Criminal evidence: principles and cases.* Belmont, CA: Wadsworth. p. 100.

5. Robinson, J. 2004. Emotion: biological fact or social construction? In *Thinking about feeling: contemporary philosophers on emotion*, edited by R. Solomon. New York: Oxford University Press. p. 29

6. De Sousa, R. 1997. *The rationality of emotion*. Cambridge, MA: MIT Press. p. xv.

7. Ibid., p. 182.

8. Dolan, R. J. 2002. Emotion, cognition, and behavior. *Science* 298 (5596):1191–4.

9. Ibid.

10. James, W. 1884. What is an emotion? *Mind* 9 (34):188–205.

11. Ekman, P. 2003. Biological and cultural contributions to body and facial movement in the expression of emotions. In *What is an emotion?*, edited by R. Solomon. New York: Oxford University Press. p. 121.

12. Ekman, P., E. R. Sorenson, and W. V. Friesen. 1969. Pan-cultural elements in facial displays of emotion. *Science* 164 (875):86–8.

13. See Elliott, C. 2003. *Better than well: American medicine meets the American dream*. New York: W. W. Norton and Company. p. 71. See also American Psychiatric Association. 2000. *Diagnostic and statistical manual of mental disorders*. 4th ed., text revision ed. Washington, DC: American Psychiatric Association. pp. 452, 903.

14. Kaufman, G. 2004. *The psychology of shame: theory and treatment of shame-based syndromes*. 2nd ed. New York: Springer. p. 286.

15. Ohman, A., and J. J. Soares. 1994. "Unconscious anxiety": phobic responses to masked stimuli. *Journal of Abnormal Psychology* 103 (2):231–40.

16. Ohman, A. 2005. The role of the amygdala in human fear: automatic detection of threat. *Psychoneuroendocrinology* 30 (10):953–8.

17. Lazarus, R. S. 1994. Appraisal: the long and the short of it. In *The nature of emotion: fundamental questions*, edited by P. Ekman and R. J. Davidson. New York: Oxford University Press. p. 209-10.

18. Ibid., p. 211.

19. Ibid., p. 210.

20. Hsee, C. K., and H. C. Kunreuther. 2000. The affection effect in insurance decisions. *Journal of Risk and Uncertainty* 20 (2):141–59.

21. Ibid.

22. Ibid.

23. Frijda, N. H. 2003. Emotions are functional, most of the time. In *What is an emotion?*, edited by R. Solomon. New York: Oxford University Press.

24. Ibid., p. 133.

25. Ibid., p. 133.

26. This is Antonio Damasio's term. He defines an emotionally competent stimulus as "the object or event whose presence, actual or in mental recall, triggers the emotion." See, Damasio, A. 2004. *Looking for Spinoza: joy, sorrow and the feeling brain.* London: Vintage. p. 53.

27. James., p. 189.

28. Ibid., p. 193.

29. Ibid., p. 190.

30. Ibid., p. 190.

31. Damasio, *Looking for Spinoza*, p. 109.

32. For a comprehensive discussion of the relevant neuroanatomy, see Craig, A. D. 2002. How do you feel? Interoception: the sense of the physiological condition of the body. *Nature Reviews: Neuroscience* 3 (8):655–66.

33. Damasio, *Looking for Spinoza*, p. 101.

34. Ibid., p. 148.

35. Strictly, while James holds emotion to be the feeling of bodily changes, Damasio describes the bodily changes, independent of feelings, as the emotion. On Damasio's account, emotion can occur without conscious feeling states.

36. Ibid., p. 53.

37. Ibid., p. 140.

38. Damasio, A. 1994. *Descartes' error.* New York: Penguin. p. 34.

39. Ibid., p. 193.

40. Bechara, A., H. Damasio, D. Tranel, and A. R. Damasio. 1997. Deciding advantageously before knowing the advantageous strategy. *Science* 275 (5304):1293–5.

41. Damasio, *Looking for Spinoza*, p. 147.

42. Ibid., p. 109.

43. Maia, T. V., and J. L. McClelland. 2004. A reexamination of the evidence for the SMH: what participants really know in the Iowa Gambling Task. *Proceedings of the National Academy of Sciences USA* 101 (45):16075–80.

44. van't Wout, M., R. S. Kahn, A. G. Sanfey, and A. Aleman. 2006. Affective state and decision-making in the Ultimatum Game. *Experimental Brain Research* 169 (4):564–8.

45. Dunn, B. D., T. Dalgleish, and A. D. Lawrence. 2006. The somatic marker hypothesis: a critical evaluation. *Neuroscience and Biobehavioral Reviews* 30 (2):239–71.

46. Ibid.

47. Elliot, R. 1998. A model of emotion-driven choice. *Journal of Marketing Management* 14: 95–108.

48. De Houwer, J., S. Thomas, and F. Baeyens. 2001. Associative learning of likes and dislikes: a review of 25 years of research on human evaluative conditioning. *Psychological Bulletin* 127 (6):853–69.

49. Gibson, B. 2008. Can evaluative conditioning change attitudes toward mature brands? New evidence from the implicit association test. *Journal of Consumer Research* 35:178–88.

50. Friese, M., M. Wanke, and H. Plessner. 2006. Implicit consumer preferences and their influence on product choice. *Psychology and Marketing* 23 (9):727–40.

51. Slovic, P., M. Finucane, E. Peters, and D. G. MacGregor. 2002. The affect heuristic. In *Heuristics and biases: the psychology of intuitive judgment*, edited by T. Gilovich, D. Griffin, and D. Kahneman. Cambridge: Cambridge University Press.

52. Ibid., p. 400.

53. For a description, see Gohm, C. L., and G. L. Clore. 2002. Affect as information: an individual differences approach. In *The wisdom in feelings: processes underlying emotional intelligence*, edited by L. Feldman Barrett and P. Salovey. New York: Guilford Press.

54. Pham, M. T. 2004. The logic of feeling. *Journal of Consumer Psychology* 14 (4):360–9.

55. Mayer, J. D., P. Salovey, D. R. Caruso, and G. Sitarenios. 2001. Emotional intelligence as a standard intelligence. *Emotion* 1 (3):232–42.

56. Mayer, J. D., P. Salovey, and D. R. Caruso. 2008. Emotional intelligence: new ability or eclectic traits? *American Psychologist* 63 (6):503–17.

57. Frijda, N.H., and B. Mesquita. 2000. Beliefs through emotions. In *Emotions and beliefs: how feelings influence thoughts,* edited by N. H. Frijda, A. S. R. Manstead and S. Bem. Cambridge: Cambridge University Press. p. 55.

58. See, for example, Guyatt, G. H., R. B. Haynes, R. Z. Jaeschke, D. J. Cook, L. Green, C. D. Naylor, M. C. Wilson, and W. S. Richardson. 2000. Users' guides to the medical literature: XXV. Evidence-based medicine: principles for applying the users' guides to patient care. Evidence-Based Medicine Working Group. *Journal of the American Medical Association* 284 (10):1290–6.

59. Scharwz, N., and G. L. Clore. 1983. Mood, misattribution, and judgments of well-being: informative and directive functions of affective states. *Journal of Personality and Social Psychology* 45 (3):513–23.

60. Slovic, Finucane, Peters, and MacGregor, p. 417.

61. Finucane, M. L., A. Alhakami, P. Slovic, and S. M. Johnson. 2000. The affect heuristic in judgments of risks and benefits. *Journal of Behavioral Decision Making* 13:1–17.

62. Slovic, Finucane, Peters, and MacGregor, pp. 417–8.

63. Slovic, P. 2001. Cigarette smokers: rational actors or rational fools? In *Smoking: risk, perception, and policy*, edited by P. Slovic. Thousand Oaks, CA: Sage. p. 121.

64. Gilbert, P. 1998. The evolved basis and adaptive functions of cognitive distortions. *British Journal of Medical Psychology* 71 (Pt. 4):447–63.

65. Tversky, A., and D. Kahneman. 1974. Judgment under uncertainty: heuristics and biases. *Science* 185 (4157):1124–31.

66. Pham, M.T. 1998. Representativeness, relevance, and the use of feelings in decision-making. *Journal of Consumer Research* 25 (2):144–59.

67. Tiedens, L. Z., and S. Linton. 2001. Judgment under emotional certainty and uncertainty: the effects of specific emotions on information processing. *Journal of Personality and Social Psychology* 81 (6):973–88.

68. Lerner, J. S., and L. Z. Tiedens. 2006. Portrait of the angry decision maker: how appraisal tendencies shape anger's influence on cognition. *Journal of Behavioral Decision Making* 19:115–37.

69. Tiedens and Linton.

Chapter 4

1. American Psychiatric Association, *Diagnostic and statistical manual of mental disorders*, p. 349.

2. Ibid., p. 2.

3. Horwitz, A. V., and J. C. Wakefield. 2007. *The loss of sadness: how psychiatry transformed normal sorrow into depressive disorder.* Oxford; New York: Oxford University Press. p. 6.

4. Beck, A. T., J. A. Rush, B. F. Shaw, and G. Emery. 1979. *Cognitive therapy of depression.* New York: Guilford Press.

5. Clark, D. A., A. T. Beck, and B. A. Alford. 1999. *Scientific foundations of cognitive theory of depression.* New York: John Wiley.

6. Ellis and Smith.

7. Butler, A. C., J. E. Chapman, E. M. Forman, and A. T. Beck. 2006. The empirical status of cognitive–behavioral therapy: a review of meta-analyses. *Clinical Psychology Review* 26 (1):17–31.

8. DeRubeis, R. J., G. J. Siegle, and S. D. Hollon. 2008. Cognitive therapy versus medication for depression: treatment outcomes and neural mechanisms. *Nature Reviews: Neuroscience* 9 (10):788–96.

9. Andersen, S. M., L. A. Spielman, and J. A. Bargh. 2002. Future-event schemas and certainty about the future: automaticity in the depressive's future event predictions. *Journal of Personality and Social Psychology* 63 (5):711–23.

10. Beck, Rush, Shaw, and Emery, p. 11.

11. CBT will be discussed in detail in chapter 5.

12. Watkins, P. C., K. Vache, S. P. Verney, S. Muller, and A. Mathews. 1996. Unconscious mood-congruent memory bias in depression. *Journal of Abnormal Psychology* 105 (1):34–41.

13. Mathews, A., and C. MacLeod. 2005. Cognitive vulnerability to emotional disorders. *Annual Review of Clinical Psychology* 1:167–95.

14. Koster, E. H., R. De Raedt, E. Goeleven, E. Franck, and G. Crombez. 2005. Mood-congruent attentional bias in dysphoria: maintained attention to and impaired disengagement from negative information. *Emotion* 5 (4):446–55.

15. Gotlib, I. H., E. Krasnoperova, D. N. Yue, and J. Joormann. 2004. Attentional biases for negative interpersonal stimuli in clinical depression. *Journal of Abnormal Psychology* 113 (1):121–35.

16. Kahneman received the Nobel Prize in Economic Sciences in 2002 in recognition of his research into human judgment and decision making under uncertainty.

17. Tversky and Kahneman.

18. Ibid.

19. Ibid.

20. Taylor, S. 1982. The availability bias in social perception and interaction. In *Judgment under uncertainty: heuristics and biases*, edited by D. Kahneman, P. Slovic, and A. Tversky. Cambridge; New York: Cambridge University Press.

21. MacLeod, C., and L. Campbell. 1992. Memory accessibility and probability judgments: an experimental evaluation of the availability heuristic. *Journal of Personality and Social Psychology* 63 (6):890–902.

22. Ibid.

23. Ibid.

24. MacLeod, A. K., P. Tata, J. Kentish, F. Carroll, and E. Hunter. 1997. Anxiety, depression, and explanation-based pessimism for future positive and negative events. *Clinical Psychology and Psychotherapy* 4 (1):15–24.

25. Kahneman, D., and A. Tversky. 1982. The simulation heuristic. In *Judgment under uncertainty: heuristics and biases*, edited by D. Kahneman, P. Slovic, and A. Tversky. Cambridge; New York: Cambridge University Press.

26. MacLeod, Tata, Kentish, Carroll, and Hunter.

27. Vaughn, L., and G. Weary. 2002. Roles of the availability of explanations, feelings of ease, and dysphoria in judgments about the future. *Journal of Social and Clinical Psychology* 21 (6):686–704.

28. Koster, E. H., E. Fox, and C. MacLeod. 2009. Introduction to the special section on cognitive bias modification in emotional disorders. *Journal of Abnormal Psychology* 118 (1):1–4.

29. Mathews and MacLeod.

30. Alloy, L. B., and L. Y. Abramson. 1979. Judgment of contingency in depressed and nondepressed students: sadder but wiser? *Journal of Experimental Psychology: General* 108 (4):441–85.

31. Kendler, Karkowski, and Prescott.

32. Moore, M. T., and D. M. Fresco. 2007. Depressive realism and attributional style: implications for individuals at risk for depression. *Behavior Therapy* 38 (2):144–54.

33. MacLeod, Tata, Kentish, Carroll, and Hunter.

34. MacLeod and Campbell.

35. Andersen, Spielman, and Bargh.

36. Abramson, L. Y., G. I. Metalsky, and L. B. Alloy. 1989. Hopelessness depression: a theory-based subtype of depression. *Psychological Review* 96 (2):358–72.

37. Fu, T., W. Koutstaal, C. H. Y. Fu, L. Poon, and A. J. Cleare. 2005. Depression, confidence and decision: evidence against depressive realism. *Journal of Psychopathology and Behavioral Assessment* 27 (4):243–52.

38. Dunning, D., and A. L. Story. 1991. Depression, realism, and the overconfidence effect: are the sadder wiser when predicting future actions and events? *Journal of Personality and Social Psychology* 61 (4):521–32.

39. Carson, R. C., S. D. Hollon, and R. C. Shelton. 2010. Depressive realism and clinical depression. *Behavior Research and Therapy* 48 (4):257–65.

40. Teasdale, J. D., R. G. Moore, H. Hayhurst, M. Pope, S. Williams, and Z. V. Segal. 2002. Metacognitive awareness and prevention of relapse in depression: empirical evidence. *Journal of Consulting and Clinical Psychology* 70 (2):275–87.

41. Ibid.

42. Kuyken, W., S. Byford, R. S. Taylor, E. Watkins, E. Holden, K. White, B. Barrett, R. Byng, A. Evans, E. Mullan, and J. D. Teasdale. 2008. Mindfulness-based cognitive therapy to prevent relapse in recurrent depression. *Journal of Consulting and Clinical Psychology* 76 (6):966–78.

43. Clark, Beck, and Alford, p. 292.

44. Kendler, Karkowski, and Prescott.

45. Ibid.

46. Kessler, R. C. 1997. The effects of stressful life events on depression. *Annual Review of Psychology* 48:191–214.

47. Hammen, C. 2005. Stress and depression. *Annual Review of Clinical Psychology* 1:293–319.

48. Allen, N. B., and P. B. Badcock. 2003. The social risk hypothesis of depressed mood: evolutionary, psychosocial, and neurobiological perspectives. *Psychological Bulletin* 129 (6):887–913.

49. Farmer, A. E., and P. McGuffin. 2003. Humiliation, loss and other types of life events and difficulties: a comparison of depressed subjects, healthy controls and their siblings. *Psychological Medicine* 33 (7):1169–75.

50. Post, R. M. 1992. Transduction of psychosocial stress into the neurobiology of recurrent affective disorder. *American Journal of Psychiatry* 149 (8):999–1010.

51. Stroud, C. B., J. Davila, and A. Moyer. 2008. The relationship between stress and depression in first onsets versus recurrences: a meta-analytic review. *Journal of Abnormal Psychology* 117 (1):206–13.

52. Kendler, K. S., L. M. Thornton, and C. O. Gardner. 2000. Stressful life events and previous episodes in the etiology of major depression in women: an evaluation of the "kindling" hypothesis. *American Journal of Psychiatry* 157 (8):1243–51.

53. For a review, see Monroe, S. M., and K. L. Harkness. 2005. Life stress, the "kindling" hypothesis, and the recurrence of depression: considerations from a life stress perspective. *Psychological Review* 112 (2):417–45.

54. American Psychiatric Association, *Diagnostic and statistical manual of mental disorders*, p. 420.

55. Mitchell, P. B., G. B. Parker, G. L. Gladstone, K. Wilhelm, and M. P. Austin. 2003. Severity of stressful life events in first and subsequent episodes of depression: the relevance of depressive subtype. *Journal of Affective Disorders* 73 (3):245–52.

56. Brown, G. W., T. O. Harris, and C. Hepworth. 1994. Life events and endogenous depression: A puzzle reexamined. *Archives of General Psychiatry* 51 (7):525–34.

57. Harkness, K. L., and S. M. Monroe. 2006. Severe melancholic depression is more vulnerable than non-melancholic depression to minor precipitating life events. *Journal of Affective Disorders* 91 (2–3):257–63.

58. Thase, M. E., and E. S. Friedman. 1999. Is psychotherapy an effective treatment for melancholia and other severe depressive states? *Journal of Affective Disorders* 54 (1–2):1–19.

59. Luty, S. E., J. D. Carter, J. M. McKenzie, A. M. Rae, C. M. Frampton, R. T. Mulder, and P. R. Joyce. 2007. Randomized controlled trial of interpersonal psychotherapy and cognitive–behavioral therapy for depression. *British Journal of Psychiatry* 190:496–502.

60. Black Dog Institute. 2009. *Fact sheet: types of depression* 2009 [cited April 22, 2009]. Available from <http://www.blackdoginstitute.org.au/docs/TypesofDepression.pdf>.

61. Gould, E., P. Tanapat, B. S. McEwen, G. Flugge, and E. Fuchs. 1998. Proliferation of granule cell precursors in the dentate gyrus of adult monkeys is diminished by stress. *Proceedings of the National Academy of Sciences USA* 95 (6):3168–71.

62. Shah, P. J., K. P. Ebmeier, M. F. Glabus, and G. M. Goodwin. 1998. Cortical gray matter reductions associated with treatment-resistant chronic unipolar depression: controlled magnetic resonance imaging study. *British Journal of Psychiatry* 172:527–32.

63. Videbech, P., and B. Ravnkilde. 2004. Hippocampal volume and depression: a meta-analysis of MRI studies. *American Journal of Psychiatry* 161 (11):1957–66.

64. Nestler, E. J., M. Barrot, R. J. DiLeone, A. J. Eisch, S. J. Gold, and L. M. Monteggia. 2002. Neurobiology of depression. *Neuron* 34 (1):13–25.

65. Sapolsky, R. M. 2004. Is impaired neurogenesis relevant to the affective symptoms of depression? *Biological Psychiatry* 56 (3):137–9.

66. Nestler, Barrot, DiLeone, Eisch, Gold, and Monteggia.

67. van Eck, M., H. Berkhof, N. Nicolson, and J. Sulon. 1996. The effects of perceived stress, traits, mood states, and stressful daily events on salivary cortisol. *Psychosomatic Medicine* 58 (5):447–58.

68. Sayal, K., S. Checkley, M. Rees, C. Jacobs, T. Harris, A. Papadopoulos, and L. Poon. 2002. Effects of social support during weekend leave on cortisol and depression ratings: a pilot study. *Journal of Affective Disorders* 71 (1–3):153–7.

69. Sher, L. 2004. Daily hassles, cortisol, and the pathogenesis of depression. *Medical Hypotheses* 62 (2):198–202.

70. van Praag, H. M. 2004. Can stress cause depression? *Progress in Neuro-Psychopharmacology and Biological Psychiatry* 28 (5):891–907.

71. Reid, I. C., and C. A. Stewart. 2001. How antidepressants work: new perspectives on the pathophysiology of depressive disorder. *British Journal of Psychiatry* 178:299–303.

72. Belmaker, R. H., and G. Agam. 2008. Major depressive disorder. *New England Journal of Medicine* 358 (1):55–68.

73. Duman, R. S., and L. M. Monteggia. 2006. A neurotrophic model for stress-related mood disorders. *Biological Psychiatry* 59 (12):1116–27.

74. Ibid.

75. In this study, an example of a questionnaire item denoting a disturbed family environment was "Family members would get so angry sometimes that they would throw things or hit each other."

76. Kendler, K. S., C. O. Gardner, and C. A. Prescott. 2002. Toward a comprehensive developmental model for major depression in women. *American Journal of Psychiatry* 159 (7):1133–45.

77. Kendler, K. S., C. O. Gardner, and C. A. Prescott. 2006. Toward a comprehensive developmental model for major depression in men. *American Journal of Psychiatry* 163 (1):115–24.

78. Lumley, M. N., and K. L. Harkness. 2007. Specificity in the relations among childhood adversity, early maladaptive schemas, and symptom profiles in adolescent depression. *Cognitive Therapy and Research* 31:639–57.

79. Kercher, A., and R. M. Rapee. 2009. A test of a cognitive diathesis–stress generation pathway in early adolescent depression. *Journal of Abnormal Child Psychology* 37 (6):845–55.

80. Serotonin is also known as 5-hydroxytryptamine, or 5-HT.

81. Kramer, P. D. 2005. *Against depression*. New York: Viking. p. 130.

82. Caspi, A., K. Sugden, T. E. Moffitt, A. Taylor, I. W. Craig, H. Harrington, J. McClay, J. Mill, J. Martin, A. Braithwaite, and R. Poulton. 2003. Influence of life stress on depression: moderation by a polymorphism in the 5-HTT gene. *Science* 301 (5631):386–9.

83. Kendler, K. S., J. W. Kuhn, J. Vittum, C. A. Prescott, and B. Riley. 2005. The interaction of stressful life events and a serotonin transporter polymorphism in the prediction of episodes of major depression: a replication. *Archives of General Psychiatry* 62 (5):529–35.

84. Anguelova, M., C. Benkelfat, and G. Turecki. 2003. A systematic review of association studies investigating genes coding for serotonin receptors and the serotonin transporter: I. Affective disorders. *Molecular Psychiatry* 8 (6):574–91.

85. Risch, N., R. Herrell, T. Lehner, K. Y. Liang, L. Eaves, J. Hoh, A. Griem, M. Kovacs, J. Ott, and K. R. Merikangas. 2009. Interaction between the serotonin transporter gene (5-HTTLPR), stressful life events, and risk of depression: a meta-analysis. *Journal of the American Medical Association* 301 (23):2462–71.

86. Kendler, Karkowski, and Prescott.

87. Ibid.

88. Rozanski, A., J. A. Blumenthal, K. W. Davidson, P. G. Saab, and L. Kubzansky. 2005. The epidemiology, pathophysiology, and management of psychosocial risk factors in cardiac practice: the emerging field of behavioral cardiology. *Journal of the American College of Cardiology* 45 (5):637–51.

89. Reid, G. J., P. H. Seidelin, W. J. Kop, M. J. Irvine, B. H. Strauss, R. P. Nolan, H. K. Lau, and E. L. Yeo. 2009. Mental-stress-induced platelet activation among patients with coronary artery disease. *Psychosomatic Medicine* 71 (4):438–45.

90. Matschinger, H., and M. C. Angermeyer. 1996. Lay beliefs about the causes of mental disorders: a new methodological approach. *Social Psychiatry and Psychiatric Epidemiology* 31 (6):309–15.

91. Angermeyer, M. C., and H. Matschinger. 2003. Public beliefs about schizophrenia and depression: similarities and differences. *Social Psychiatry and Psychiatric Epidemiology* 38 (9):526–34.

92. Lauber, C., L. Falcato, C. Nordt, and W. Rossler. 2003. Lay beliefs about causes of depression. *Acta Psychiatrica Scandinavica: Supplementum* (418):96–9.

93. Blumner, K. H., and S. C. Marcus. 2009. Changing perceptions of depression: ten-year trends from the General Social Survey. *Psychiatric Services* 60 (3):306–12.

94. Srinivasan, J., N. L. Cohen, and S. V. Parikh. 2003. Patient attitudes regarding causes of depression: implications for psychoeducation. *Canadian Journal of Psychiatry* 48 (7):493–5.

95. Brown, C., J. Dunbar-Jacob, D. R. Palenchar, K. J. Kelleher, R. D. Bruehlman, S. Sereika, and M. E. Thase. 2001. Primary care patients' personal illness models for depression: a preliminary investigation. *Family Practice* 18 (3):314–20.

96. Mental Health America of Indiana. 2010. *Depression: depression and bipolar support alliance* [cited February 1, 2010]. Available from <http://www.mentalhealthassociation.com/IDMDA.htm>.

97. Deacon, B. J., and G. L. Baird. 2009. The chemical imbalance explanation of depression: reducing blame at what cost? *Journal of Social and Clinical Psychology* 28 (4):415–35.

98. Ibid.

99. Ibid.

100. Harkness and Monroe.

101. Australian Institute of Health and Welfare, p. 44.

102. Ibid., p. 46.

103. Ibid., p. 48

104. Australian Institute of Health and Welfare.

105. Ibid., p. 40.

106. National Center for Health Statistics.

107. Stagnitti. Antidepressants prescribed by medical doctors in office based and outpatient settings by specialty for the U.S. civilian noninstitutionalized population, 2002 and 2005.

108. Stagnitti, M. N. 2004. Top 10 outpatient prescription medicines ranked by utilization and expenditures for the U.S. community population 2002. Rockville, MD: Agency for Healthcare Research and Quality.

109. Robinson, W. D., J. A. Geske, L. A. Prest, and R. Barnacle. 2005. Depression treatment in primary care. *Journal of the American Board of Family Practice* 18 (2):79–86.

110. Olfson, M., S. C. Marcus, B. Druss, L. Elinson, T. Tanielian, and H. A. Pincus. 2002. National trends in the outpatient treatment of depression. *Journal of the American Medical Association* 287 (2):203–9.

111. France, C. M., P. H. Lysaker, and R. P. Robinson. 2007. The "chemical imbalance" explanation for depression: origins, lay endorsement, and clinical implications. *Professional Psychology: Research and Practice* 38 (4):411–20.

112. Leykin, Y., R. J. DeRubeis, R. C. Shelton, and J. D. Amsterdam. 2007. Changes in patients' beliefs about the causes of their depression following successful treatment. *Cognitive Therapy and Research* 31:437–49.

113. Thomas-MacLean, R., and J. M. Stoppard. 2004. Physicians' constructions of depression: inside/outside the boundaries of medicalization. *Health (London)* 8 (3):275–93.

114. Ibid.

115. Schreiber, R., and G. Hartrick. 2002. Keeping it together: how women use the biomedical explanatory model to manage the stigma of depression. *Issues in Mental Health Nursing* 23 (2):91–105.

116. Ibid.

117. Ellis and Smith.

118. Australian Institute of Health and Welfare, p. 44.

119. Wolf, N. J., and D. R. Hopko. 2008. Psychosocial and pharmacological interventions for depressed adults in primary care: a critical review. *Clinical Psychology Review* 28 (1):131–61.

120. Rogers, A., C. May, and D. Oliver. 2001. Experiencing depression, experiencing the depressed: The separate worlds of patients and doctors. *Journal of Mental Health* 10 (3):317–33.

121. Pollock, K., and J. Grime. 2003. GPs' perspectives on managing time in consultations with patients suffering from depression: a qualitative study. *Family Practice* 20 (3):262–9.

122. Ibid.

123. Mynors-Wallis, L. M., D. H. Gath, A. Day, and F. Baker. 2000. Randomized controlled trial of problem solving treatment, antidepressant medication, and combined treatment for major depression in primary care. *British Medical Journal* 320 (7226):26–30.

124. Alloy, L. B., A. J. Lipman, and L. Y. Abramson. 1992. Attributional style as a vulnerability factor for depression: validation by past history of mood disorders. *Cognitive Therapy and Research* 16 (4):391–407.

125. Abramson, Metalsky, and Alloy.

126. Kwon, P., and J. P. Laurenceau. 2002. A longitudinal study of the hopelessness theory of depression: testing the diathesis–stress model within a differential reactivity and exposure framework. *Journal of Clinical Psychology* 58 (10):1305–21.

127. Hankin, B. L. 2008. Cognitive vulnerability–stress model of depression during adolescence: investigating depressive symptom specificity in a multi-wave prospective study. *Journal of Abnormal Child Psychology* 36 (7):999–1014.

128. Jacobs, R. H., M. A. Reinecke, J. K. Gollan, and P. Kane. 2008. Empirical evidence of cognitive vulnerability for depression among children and adolescents: a cognitive science and developmental perspective. *Clinical Psychology Review* 28 (5):759–82.

129. The role of problem-oriented treatments in depression is examined in detail in chapter 6.

130. Persons, J. B., and J. Miranda. 1992. Cognitive theories of vulnerability to depression: reconciling negative evidence. *Cognitive Therapy and Research* 16 (4):485–502.

131. Gladstone, G., and G. Parker. 2001. Depressogenic cognitive schemas: enduring beliefs or mood state artifacts? *Australian and New Zealand Journal of Psychiatry* 35 (2):210–6.

132. Ball, H. A., P. McGuffin, and A. E. Farmer. 2008. Attributional style and depression. *British Journal of Psychiatry* 192 (4):275–8.

133. Otto, M. W., B. A. Teachman, L. S. Cohen, C. N. Soares, A. F. Vitonis, and B. L. Harlow. 2007. Dysfunctional attitudes and episodes of major depression: Predictive validity and temporal stability in never-depressed, depressed, and recovered women. *Journal of Abnormal Psychology* 116 (3):475–83.

Chapter 5

1. Roth, A., and P. Fonagy. 1996. *What works for whom? A critical review of psychotherapy research.* New York: Guilford Press. p. 5.

2. Ibid. p. 5.

3. DeRubeis, Siegle, and Hollon.

4. MBCT is an intervention specifically for relapse prevention. See, for example, Kuyken, Byford, Taylor, Watkins, Holden, White, Barrett, Byng, Evans, Mullan, and Teasdale.

5. Luty, Carter, McKenzie, Rae, Frampton, Mulder, and Joyce.

6. Bell, A. C., and T. J. D'Zurilla. 2009. Problem-solving therapy for depression: a meta-analysis. *Clinical Psychology Review* 29 (4):348–53.

7. Andersen, Spielman, and Bargh.

8. Wenze, S. J., K. C. Gunthert, and N. R. Forand. 2007. Influence of dysphoria on positive and negative cognitive reactivity to daily mood fluctuations. *Behavior Research and Therapy* 45 (5):915–27.

9. Otto, Teachman, Cohen, Soares, Vitonis, and Harlow.

10. Beck, A. T., and B. A. Alford. 2009. *Depression: causes and treatment*. Philadelphia: University of Pennsylvania Press. p. 199.

11. American Psychiatric Association, *Diagnostic and statistical manual of mental disorders*.

12. Beck, A. T., and M.E. Weishaar. 2008. Cognitive therapy. In *Current psychotherapies*, edited by R. J. Corsini and D. Wedding. Belmont, CA: Thomson Brooks Cole. p. 264.

13. Ibid., p. 285.

14. Hayes, B., and B. Hesketh. 1989. Attribution theory, judgmental biases, and cognitive behavior modification: prospects and problems. *Cognitive Therapy and Research* 13 (3):211–230.

15. Hollon, S. D., and R. J. Derubeis. 2009. Mediating the effects of cognitive therapy for depression. *Cognitive Behaviour Therapy* 38 (S1):43–47.

16. Hirt, E. R., and K. D. Markman. 1995. Multiple explanation: a consider-an-alternative strategy for debiasing judgments. *Journal of Personality and Social Psychology* 69 (6):1069–86.

17. This scenario was originally used in Anderson, C. A., M. R. Lepper, and L. Ross. 1980. Perseverance of social theories: the role of explanation in the persistence of discredited information. *Journal of Personality and Social Psychology* 39 (6):1037–49.

18. Ibid.

19. MacLeod, Tata, Kentish, Carroll, and Hunter.

20. Chapter 4, section 4.2.2.

21. Chapter 4, section 4.2.2.

22. Bentz, B. G., D. A. Williamson, and S. F. Franks. 2004. Debiasing of pessimistic judgments associated with anxiety. *Journal of Psychopathology and Behavioral Assessment* 26 (3):173–80.

23. Ibid.

24. Tang, T. Z., R. J. Derubeis, S. D. Hollon, J. Amsterdam, and R. Shelton. 2007. Sudden gains in cognitive therapy of depression and depression relapse/recurrence. *Journal of Consulting and Clinical Psychology* 75 (3):404–8.

25. Ibid.

26. Tang, T. Z., and R. J. DeRubeis. 1999. Sudden gains and critical sessions in cognitive–behavioral therapy for depression. *Journal of Consulting and Clinical Psychology* 67 (6):894–904.

27. Ibid.

28. Beck, Rush, Shaw, and Emery, p. 158.

29. Ibid.

30. Teasdale, J. D., Z. Segal, and J. M. Williams. 1995. How does cognitive therapy prevent depressive relapse and why should attentional control (mindfulness) training help? *Behavior Research and Therapy* 33 (1):25–39.

31. Ibid.

32. Ibid.

33. Teasdale, J. D., R. G. Moore, H. Hayhurst, M. Pope, S. Williams, and Z. V. Segal. 2002. Metacognitive awareness and prevention of relapse in depression: empirical evidence. *Journal of Consulting and Clinical Psychology* 70 (2):275–87.

34. Rumination is discussed in detail in chapter 6, section 6.2. See also Nolen-Hoeksema, S. 1991. Responses to depression and their effects on the duration of depressive episodes. *Journal of Abnormal Psychology* 100 (4):569–82.

35. Kabat-Zinn, J. 1994. *Wherever you go, there you are: mindfulness meditation in everyday life.* New York: Hyperion. p. 4, cited in Allen, N. B., R. Chambers, and W. Knight. 2006. Mindfulness-based psychotherapies: a review of conceptual foundations, empirical evidence and practical considerations. *Australian and New Zealand Journal of Psychiatry* 40 (4):285–94.

36. Allen, Chambers, and Knight.

37. See Finucane, A., and S. W. Mercer. 2006. An exploratory mixed methods study of the acceptability and effectiveness of mindfulness-based cognitive therapy for patients with active depression and anxiety in primary care. *BMC Psychiatry* 6 (14); Kabat-Zinn, J. 1990. *Full Catastrophe Living; The program of the Stress Reduction Clinic at the University of Massachusetts Medical Center.* Reprint ed. New York: Delta; Ma, S. H., and J. D. Teasdale. 2004. Mindfulness-based cognitive therapy for depression: replication and exploration of differential relapse prevention effects. *Journal of Consulting and Clinical Psychology* 72 (1):31–40; Teasdale, Moore, Hayhurst, Pope, Williams, and Segal.

38. Beck, Rush, Shaw, and Emery, p. 117.

39. Ibid., p. 128.

40. Hollon and DeRubeis.

41. Beck, Rush, Shaw, and Emery, p. 159.

42. Berton, O., and E. J. Nestler. 2006. New approaches to antidepressant drug discovery: beyond monoamines. *Nature reviews: Neuroscience* 7 (2):137–51.

43. Harmer, C. J., S. A. Hill, M. J. Taylor, P. J. Cowen, and G. M. Goodwin. 2003. Toward a neuropsychological theory of antidepressant drug action: increase in

positive emotional bias after potentiation of norepinephrine activity. *American Journal of Psychiatry* 160 (5):990–2.

44. Harmer, C. J., N. C. Shelley, P. J. Cowen, and G. M. Goodwin. 2004. Increased positive versus negative affective perception and memory in healthy volunteers following selective serotonin and norepinephrine reuptake inhibition. *American Journal of Psychiatry* 161 (7):1256–63.

45. These largely correspond to Paul Ekman's list of the six facial expressions that are near-universally recognized. See Ekman, Sorenson, and Friesen.

46. Harmer, Shelley, Cowen, and Goodwin.

47. Harmer, Hill, Taylor, Cowen, and Goodwin.

48. Harmer, C. J., U. O'Sullivan, E. Favaron, R. Massey-Chase, R. Ayres, A. Reinecke, G. M. Goodwin, and P. J. Cowen. 2009. Effect of acute antidepressant administration on negative affective bias in depressed patients. *American Journal of Psychiatry* 166 (10):1178–84.

49. Tranter, R., D. Bell, P. Gutting, C. Harmer, D. Healy, and I. M. Anderson. 2009. The effect of serotonergic and noradrenergic antidepressants on face emotion processing in depressed patients. *Journal of Affective Disorders* 118 (1–3):87–93.

50. Harmer, C. J., G. M. Goodwin, and P. J. Cowen. 2009. Why do antidepressants take so long to work? A cognitive neuropsychological model of antidepressant drug action. *British Journal of Psychiatry* 195 (2):102–8.

51. Ibid.

52. Harmer, Shelley, Cowen, and Goodwin.

53. Knutson, B., O. M. Wolkowitz, S. W. Cole, T. Chan, E. A. Moore, R. C. Johnson, J. Terpstra, R. A. Turner, and V. I. Reus. 1998. Selective alteration of personality and social behavior by serotonergic intervention. *American Journal of Psychiatry* 155 (3):373–9.

54. Ibid.

55. Simmons, J. G., N. B. Allen, F. K. Judd, and T. R. Norman. The effects of fluoxetine on mood and emotional responsiveness. Personal communication, Professor Nicholas Allen, School of Psychological Sciences, University of Melbourne, Australia.

56. Opbroek, A., P. L. Delgado, C. Laukes, C. McGahuey, J. Katsanis, F. A. Moreno, and R. Manber. 2002. Emotional blunting associated with SSRI-induced sexual dysfunction: do SSRIs inhibit emotional responses? *International Journal of Neuropsychopharmacology* 5 (2):147–51.

57. Ibid.

58. Price, J., V. Cole, and G. M. Goodwin. 2009. Emotional side-effects of selective serotonin reuptake inhibitors: qualitative study. *British Journal of Psychiatry* 195 (3):211–7.

59. Ibid.

60. This account has some parallels with Martin Seligman's concept, "flexible optimism." Seligman argues optimism to be an important trait, particularly in conferring resilience to adversity, but that pessimism too has utility, especially in alerting individuals to events that threaten their interests. "What we want is not blind optimism but flexible optimism—optimism with its eyes open. We must be able to use pessimism's keen sense of reality when we need it, but without having to dwell in its dark shadows." Seligman, M. E. P. 2006. *Learned optimism: how to change your mind and your life*. 1st Vintage Books ed. New York: Vintage Books. p. 292.

61. Drevets, W. C. 2001. Neuroimaging and neuropathological studies of depression: implications for the cognitive-emotional features of mood disorders. *Current Opinion in Neurobiology* 11 (2):240–9.

62. Drevets, W. C. 2003. Neuroimaging abnormalities in the amygdala in mood disorders. *Annals of the New York Academy of Sciences* 985:420–44.

63. Harmer, C. J., C. E. Mackay, C. B. Reid, P. J. Cowen, and G. M. Goodwin. 2006. Antidepressant drug treatment modifies the neural processing of nonconscious threat cues. *Biological Psychiatry* 59 (9):816–20.

64. Sheline, Y. I., D. M. Barch, J. M. Donnelly, J. M. Ollinger, A. Z. Snyder, and M. A. Mintun. 2001. Increased amygdala response to masked emotional faces in depressed subjects resolves with antidepressant treatment: an fMRI study. *Biological Psychiatry* 50 (9):651–8.

65. DeRubeis, Siegle, and Hollon.

66. Ibid.

Chapter 6

1. McEwen, B. S. 2000. The neurobiology of stress: from serendipity to clinical relevance. *Brain Research* 886 (1–2):172–89. (Italics added.)

2. Crowe, M., and S. Luty. 2005. The process of change in interpersonal psychotherapy (IPT) for depression: a case study for the new IPT therapist. *Psychiatry* 68 (1):43–54.

3. Mynors-Wallis, L. 2005. *Problem solving treatment for anxiety and depression: a practical guide*: Oxford; New York: Oxford University Press.

4. Gaab, J., N. Blattler, T. Menzi, B. Pabst, S. Stoyer, and U. Ehlert. 2003. Randomized controlled evaluation of the effects of cognitive-behavioral stress management on

cortisol responses to acute stress in healthy subjects. *Psychoneuroendocrinology* 28 (6):767–79.

5. DeRubeis, Siegle, and Hollon.

6. Luty, Carter, McKenzie, Rae, Frampton, Mulder, and Joyce.

7. Bell and D'Zurilla.

8. See section 4.4.2.

9. Hammerfald, K., C. Eberle, M. Grau, A. Kinsperger, A. Zimmermann, U. Ehlert, and J. Gaab. 2006. Persistent effects of cognitive-behavioral stress management on cortisol responses to acute stress in healthy subjects—a randomized controlled trial. *Psychoneuroendocrinology* 31 (3):333–9.

10. Gaab, Blattler, Menzi, Pabst, Stoyer, and Ehlert.

11. Lazarus, R. S. 1993. Coping theory and research: past, present, and future. *Psychosomatic Medicine* 55 (3):234–47.

12. Reinecke, M. A. 2000. Suicide and depression. In *Cognitive-behavioral strategies in crisis intervention*, edited by F. M. Dattilio and A. Freeman. New York: Guilford Press.

13. See, for example, Gardner, B., J. Rose, O. Mason, P. Tyler, and D. Cushway. 2005. Cognitive therapy and behavioral coping in the management of work-related stress: An intervention study. *Work and Stress* 19 (2):137–52.

14. Lazarus, R. S., and S. Folkman. 1984. *Stress, appraisal, and coping*. New York: Springer.

15. See section 3.1.2.

16. Lazarus, R. S. 1999. *Stress and emotion: a new synthesis*. New York: Springer. p. 76.

17. Ibid., p. 76.

18. Ibid., p. 76.

19. Ibid., p. 76.

20. Ibid., p. 76.

21. Lazarus and Folkman, p. 141.

22. Lazarus. *Stress and emotion: a new synthesis*, p. 114.

23. Ibid., p. 114.

24. Ibid., p. 199.

25. Ibid., p. 59.

26. Lazarus and Folkman, p. 204.

27. Ibid., p. 181.

28. Meichenbaum, D. 1985. *Stress inoculation training, psychology practitioner guidebooks*. New York: Pergamon Press. p. 67.

29. For a review of recent research on stress and coping, see Folkman, S. 2009. Questions, answers, issues, and next steps in stress and coping research. *European Psychologist* 14 (1):72–7.

30. Nagase, Y., M. Uchiyama, Y. Kaneita, L. Li, T. Kaji, S. Takahashi, M. Konno, K. Mishima, T. Nishikawa, and T. Ohida. 2009. Coping strategies and their correlates with depression in the Japanese general population. *Psychiatry Research* 168 (1):57–66.

31. D'Zurilla, T. J., and A. M. Nezu. 2010. Problem-solving therapy. In *Handbook of cognitive–behavioral therapies*, edited by K. S. Dobson. New York: Guilford Press.

32. See section 2.2.1.

33. Nolen-Hoeksema.

34. Watson, P. J., and P. W. Andrews. 2002. Toward a revised evolutionary adaptationist analysis of depression: the social navigation hypothesis. *Journal of Affective Disorders* 72 (1):1–14.

35. Bishop, S. R., M. Lau, S. Shapiro, L. Carlson, N. D. Anderson, J. Carmody, Z. V. Segal, S. Abbey, M. Speca, D. Velting, and G. Devins. 2004. Mindfulness: a proposed operational definition. *Clinical Psychology: Science and Practice* 11:230–41.

36. Raes, F., D. Hermans, J. M. Williams, K. Demyttenaere, B. Sabbe, G. Pieters, and P. Eelen. 2005. Reduced specificity of autobiographical memory: a mediator between rumination and ineffective social problem-solving in major depression? *Journal of Affective Disorders* 87 (2–3):331–5.

37. Watkins, E., and S. Baracaia. 2002. Rumination and social problem-solving in depression. *Behavior Research and Therapy* 40 (10):1179–89.

38. Watkins, E., and M. Molds. 2005. Distinct modes of ruminative self-focus: Impact of abstract versus concrete rumination on problem solving in depression. *Emotion* 5 (3):319–28.

39. Martin, L. L., and A. Tesser. 2005. Toward a motivational and structural theory of ruminative thought. In *Unintended thought*, edited by J. S. Uleman and J. Bargh. New York: Guilford Press. p. 321.

40. Teasdale, J. D., Z. V. Segal, J. M. Williams, V. A. Ridgeway, J. M. Soulsby, and M. A. Lau. 2000. Prevention of relapse/recurrence in major depression by mindfulness-based cognitive therapy. *Journal of Consulting and Clinical Psychology* 68 (4):615–23.

41. See section 4.5.2.

42. See section 5.1.1.

43. Kramer, p. 187.

44. See section 4.4.2.

45. Ibid.

46. Schmidt, H. D., and R. S. Duman. 2007. The role of neurotrophic factors in adult hippocampal neurogenesis, antidepressant treatments and animal models of depressive-like behavior. *Behavioural Pharmacology* 18 (5–6):391–418.

47. Duman, R. S. 2004. Depression: a case of neuronal life and death? *Biological Psychiatry* 56 (3):140–5.

48. Warner-Schmidt, J. L., and R. S. Duman. 2006. Hippocampal neurogenesis: opposing effects of stress and antidepressant treatment. *Hippocampus* 16 (3):239–49.

49. Drevets. Neuroimaging and neuropathological studies of depression: implications for the cognitive-emotional features of mood disorders.

50. Ibid.

51. Warner-Schmidt and Duman.

52. Kramer, p. 187.

53. Ibid., p. 174.

54. Ibid., p. 185.

55. Sonino, N., G. A. Fava, P. Belluardo, M. E. Girelli, and M. Boscaro. 1993. Course of depression in Cushing's syndrome: response to treatment and comparison with Graves' disease. *Hormone Research* 39 (5–6):202–6.

56. Discussed in section 4.4.3.

57. Kramer, p. 140.

58. See section 4.4.3.

59. Kramer, p. 130.

60. Ibid., p. 148.

61. Ibid., p. 122.

62. Ibid., p. 202.

63. Nemeroff, C. B. 1998. The neurobiology of depression. *Scientific American* 278 (6):42–9.

64. Kramer, p. 56. This passage is quoted from an unnamed researcher.

65. Amado-Boccara, I., N. Gougoulis, M. F. Poirier Littre, A. Galinowski, and H. Loo. 1995. Effects of antidepressants on cognitive functions: a review. *Neuroscience and Biobehavioral Reviews* 19 (3):479–93.

66. Gorenstein, C., S. C. de Carvalho, R. Artes, R. A. Moreno, and T. Marcourakis. 2006. Cognitive performance in depressed patients after chronic use of antidepressants. *Psychopharmacology (Berl)* 185 (1):84–92.

67. Wilkinson, P. O., and I. M. Goodyer. 2008. The effects of cognitive–behavioral therapy on mood-related ruminative response style in depressed adolescents. *Child and Adolescent Psychiatry and Mental Health* 2 (1):3.

68. Wisco, B. E., and S. Nolen-Hoeksema. 2008. Ruminative response style. In *Risk factors in depression*, edited by K. S. Dobson and D. J. Dozois. Oxford: Elsevier.

69. See section 5.3.

70. Drevets. Neuroimaging and neuropathological studies of depression: implications for the cognitive-emotional features of mood disorders.

71. See section 2.2.2.

72. Faden, Beauchamp, and King, p. 307.

73. Rushton, P. J. 2004. Genetic and environmental contributions to pro-social attitudes: a twin study of social responsibility. *Proceedings of the Royal Society of London* 271:2583–5.

74. Ibid.

75. Kramer, p. 134.

76. 5-HTT is the serotonin transporter gene, detailed in chapter 4, section 4.4.3, that has been linked to depression.

77. Kramer, p. 134.

78. Ibid., p. 134.

79. Ibid., p. 148.

80. Ibid., p. 135.

81. Ibid., p. 122.

82. Ibid., p. 122.

83. See, for example, Hofmann, S. G. 2005. Perception of control over anxiety mediates the relation between catastrophic thinking and social anxiety in social phobia. *Behavior Research and Therapy* 43 (7):885–95.

84. Becker, S., and J. M. Wojtowicz. 2007. A model of hippocampal neurogenesis in memory and mood disorders. *Trends in Cognitive Sciences* 11 (2):70–6.

85. Drew, M. R., and R. Hen. 2007. Adult hippocampal neurogenesis as target for the treatment of depression. *CNS and Neurological Disorders Drug Targets* 6 (3):205–18.

86. Ibid.

87. Jacobs, B. L., H. Van Praag, and F. H. Gage. 2000. Depression and the birth and death of brain cells. *American Scientist* 88 (4):340–5.

88. Veena, J., B. N. Srikumar, T. R. Raju, and B. S. Shankaranarayana Rao. 2009. Exposure to enriched environment restores the survival and differentiation of new born cells in the hippocampus and ameliorates depressive symptoms in chronically stressed rats. *Neuroscience Letters* 455 (3):178–82.

89. Sapolsky.

90. Laperriere, A., G. H. Ironson, M. H. Antoni, H. Pomm, D. Jones, M. Ishii, D. Lydston, P. Lawrence, A. Grossman, E. Brondolo, A. Cassells, J. N. Tobin, N. Schneiderman, and S. M. Weiss. 2005. Decreased depression up to one year following CBSM+ intervention in depressed women with AIDS: the smart/EST women's project. *Journal of Health Psychology* 10 (2):223–31.

91. Hammerfald, Eberle, Grau, Kinsperger, Zimmermann, Ehlert, and Gaab.

92. Hollon, DeRubeis, Shelton, Amsterdam, Salomon, O'Reardon, Lovett, Young, Haman, Freeman, and Gallop.

Chapter 7

1. Holm, S. 2004. If you have said A, you must also say B: is this always true? *Cambridge Quarterly of Healthcare Ethics* 13 (2):179–84.

2. Royal College of Obstetricians and Gynaecologists. *RCOG statement on the paper on late termination of pregnancy published in BJOG by Habiba et al.* 2009 [cited February 22, 2010]. Available from http://www.rcog.org.uk/what-we-do/campaigning-and-opinions/statement/rcog-statement-paper-late-termination-pregnancy-publis.

3. Rachlin, K. *Transgender individuals' experiences of psychotherapy* 2002 [cited March 16, 2010]. Available from <http://www.iiav.nl/ezines/web/IJT/97-03/numbers/symposion/ijtvo06no01_03.htm>.

4. Hodgson, J., and M. Spriggs. 2005. A practical account of autonomy: why genetic counseling is especially well suited to the facilitation of informed autonomous decision making. *Journal of Genetic Counseling* 14 (2):89–97.

5. American Psychiatric Association. *Diagnostic and statistical manual of mental disorders*, p. 356.

6. The Australian Diabetes Educators Association and the Dietitians Association of Australia. 2005. *Joint statement on the role of accredited practising dietitians and diabetes educators in the delivery of nutrition and diabetes self management education services for people with diabetes* 2005 [cited September 8, 2010]. <http://www.daa .asn.au/files/DAA_A_Z/F_J/Joint%20statement%20_DAA%20and%20ADEA%20 Board%20approved_%20May%202005.pdf> (removed from site).

7. Bodenheimer, T., K. Lorig, H. Holman, and K. Grumbach. 2002. Patient self-management of chronic disease in primary care. *Journal of the American Medical Association* 288 (19):2469–75.

8. President's Commission for the Study of Ethical Problems in Medicine and Biomedical and Behavioral Research. 1983. *Deciding to forego life-sustaining treatment*. Washington, DC: U.S. Government Printing Office. p. 62.

9. de Vries, E. N., M. A. Ramrattan, S. M. Smorenburg, D. J. Gouma, and M. A. Boermeester. 2008. The incidence and nature of in-hospital adverse events: a systematic review. *Quality and Safety in Health Care* 17 (3):216–23.

10. Roth and Fonagy, p. 60.

11. Ibid., p. 60.

12. Nierenberg, A. A., and J. E. Alpert. 2000. Depressive breakthrough. *Psychiatric Clinics of North America* 23 (4):731–42.

13. Ibid.

14. Hollon, DeRubeis, Shelton, Amsterdam, Salomon, O'Reardon, Lovett, Young, Haman, Freeman, and Gallop.

15. Ibid.

16. The Hastings Center. 1996. The goals of medicine: Setting new priorities. *The Hastings Center Report* 26 (6):S1–27.

17. Ibid.

18. World Health Organization. 2009. *Constitution of the World Health Organization* [cited June 18, 2009]. Available from <http://www.searo.who.int/EN/Section898/ Section1441.htm>.

19. The Hastings Center, p. S9.

20. The Hastings Center, p. S16.

21. Stauch, M. 2000. Causal authorship and the equality principle: a defense of the acts/omissions distinction in euthanasia. *Journal of Medical Ethics* 26 (4):237–41.

22. Bayles, M. D. 1988. Professions and professionalisation. In *Ethical issues in professional life*, edited by J. C. Callahan. New York: Oxford University Press. p. 28.

23. Ibid., p. 28.

24. It is acknowledged that "off-label" medicine use is common. This is the prescription of medications for purposes other than those included in the product information. However, consistent with the claim here, guidelines affirm that any such prescribing practice should have a strong evidential basis. See Gazarian, M., M. Kelly, J. R. McPhee, L. V. Graudins, R. L. Ward, and T. J. Campbell. 2006. Off-label use of medicines: consensus recommendations for evaluating appropriateness. *The Medical Journal of Australia* 185 (10):544–8.

25. National Institute for Clinical Excellence; Ellis; American Psychiatric Association, *Practice guideline for the treatment of patients with major depressive disorder.*

26. Camenisch, P. F. 1983. *Grounding professional ethics in a pluralist society.* New York: Haven Publications. p. 31.

27. See chapter 1 for the data grounding this observation.

28. I discuss cases where beneficence might properly guide treatment recommendations in depression in section 7.3.4.

29. Haby, M. M., B. Tonge, L. Littlefield, R. Carter, and T. Vos. 2004. Cost-effectiveness of cognitive behavioral therapy and selective serotonin reuptake inhibitors for major depression in children and adolescents. *Australian and New Zealand Journal of Psychiatry* 38 (8):579–91.

30. Ibid.

31. Hollon, DeRubeis, Shelton, Amsterdam, Salomon, O'Reardon, Lovett, Young, Haman, Freeman, and Gallop.

32. Mathers, C. D., E. T. Vos, C. E. Stevenson, and S. J. Begg. 2000. The Australian Burden of Disease Study: measuring the loss of health from diseases, injuries and risk factors. *The Medical Journal of Australia* 172 (12):592–6.

33. Vos, T., J. Corry, M. M. Haby, R. Carter, and G. Andrews. 2005. Cost-effectiveness of cognitive–behavioral therapy and drug interventions for major depression. *Australian and New Zealand Journal of Psychiatry* 39 (8):683–92.

34. Medicare is a Commonwealth government program that provides health care to all Australians. Individual contributions are means assessed.

35. Antonuccio, D. O., M. Thomas, and W. G. Danton. 1997. A cost-effectiveness analysis of cognitive behavior therapy and fluoxetine (Prozac) in the treatment of depression. *Behavior Therapy* 28:187–210.

36. Pirraglia, P. A., A. B. Rosen, R. C. Hermann, N. V. Olchanski, and P. Neumann. 2004. Cost–utility analysis studies of depression management: a systematic review. *American Journal of Psychiatry* 161 (12):2155–62.

37. Ibid.

38. Layard, R. 2006. The case for psychological treatment centers. *British Medical Journal* 332 (7548):1030–2.

39. See chapter 2, section 2.3.1.

40. See chapter 4, section 4.4.2, and chapter 6, section 6.3.

41. Ellis and Smith (italics added).

Index

The Ethical Treatment of Depression

The Ethical Treatment of Depression

Autonomy through Psychotherapy

Paul Biegler

The MIT Press
Cambridge, Massachusetts
London, England

For information about special quantity discounts, please email special_sales@ mitpress.mit.edu

This book was set in Stone Sans and Stone Serif by Toppan Best-set Premedia Limited. Printed and bound in the United States of America.

Library of Congress Cataloging-in-Publication Data
Biegler, Paul, 1963–
The ethical treatment of depression : autonomy through psychotherapy / Paul Biegler.
    p. ;   cm. — (Philosophical psychopathology)
Includes bibliographical references and index.
ISBN 978-0-262-01549-3 (hardcover : alk. paper)
1. Depression, Mental—Treatment—Moral and ethical aspects. 2. Cognitive therapy—Moral and ethical aspects. 3. Autonomy (Psychology) I. Title. II. Series: Philosophical psychopathology.
[DNLM: 1. Depressive Disorder—therapy. 2. Antidepressive Agents. 3. Cognitive Therapy—ethics. 4. Personal Autonomy. WM 171]
RC537.B487   2011
174.2′968527—dc22

                                                                      2010036606

10 9 8 7 6 5 4 3 2 1